PEJMAN HAJBABAIE

Understanding Schizophrenia

First edition

This book was professionally typeset on Reedsy.
Find out more at reedsy.com

Contents

1

Chapter 1: Understanding Schizophrenia and Neuroscience of Schizophrenia

Definition and Overview

Schizophrenia is a complex and often misunderstood mental health disorder that affects how a person thinks, feels, and behaves. It is characterised by a range of symptoms, including delusions, hallucinations, disorganised thinking, and emotional dysregulation. These symptoms can significantly impair an individual's ability to function in daily life, impacting their work, relationships, and overall quality of life. Understanding schizophrenia requires a comprehensive overview of its definition, symptoms, and the various factors contributing to its onset.

The onset of schizophrenia typically occurs in late adolescence or early adulthood, although it can emerge at any age. Early diagnosis and intervention are crucial, as they can lead to better management of the disorder. Awareness of early warning signs, such as social withdrawal, changes in mood, and unusual behaviours, can enable families and friends to seek help for their loved ones before symptoms escalate. Recognising these signs is essential for timely treatment and support.

Treatment options for schizophrenia are diverse and often include a combination of medication, psychotherapy, and support services. Antipsychotic medications are commonly prescribed to manage symptoms, while therapeutic approaches such as cognitive behavioural therapy can help individuals develop coping strategies. Additionally, community support services play a vital role in providing resources and assistance for those living with schizophrenia, helping them to reintegrate into society and lead fulfilling lives.

The stigma surrounding schizophrenia is a significant barrier to understanding and acceptance of the disorder. Misconceptions and myths contribute to negative stereotypes, often leading to discrimination and social isolation for those affected. It is essential to promote awareness and education to combat these myths, fostering a more supportive environment for individuals with schizophrenia and their families.

Finally, the impact of schizophrenia extends beyond the individual, affecting family members and caregivers as well. Family support is crucial in the management of the disorder, offering emotional and practical assistance to those affected. By understanding the challenges associated with schizophrenia, families can better navigate their loved ones' needs and advocate for appropriate treatment and support. This collective effort is vital in reducing stigma and improving the overall well-being of individuals living with schizophrenia.

Neuroscience in Schizophrenia

Neuroscience has significantly advanced our understanding of schizophrenia, a complex mental disorder characterised by disruptions in thought processes, perceptions, emotional responsiveness, and social interactions. Researchers have identified various neurological anomalies associated with the disorder, including structural abnormalities in the brain. For instance, studies have shown that individuals with schizophrenia may exhibit enlarged ventricles and reduced grey matter in specific regions, which can affect cognitive functions and emotional regulation.

Understanding the neurochemical underpinnings of schizophrenia has also been a focal point of research. Neurotransmitters, particularly dopamine and glutamate, play crucial roles in the manifestation of schizophrenia symptoms. The dopamine hypothesis suggests that an overactivity of dopamine transmission may lead to positive symptoms, such as hallucinations and delusions, while glutamatergic dysfunction has been linked to negative symptoms and cognitive deficits. This knowledge has led to the development of antipsychotic medications that target these neurotransmitter systems, offering hope for symptom management.

Moreover, recent advances in neuroimaging techniques have allowed scientists to observe the brain's structure and activity in greater detail than ever before. Functional MRI (fMRI) and positron emission tomography (PET) scans have revealed alterations in brain connectivity and activity patterns in individuals with schizophrenia. These findings offer insights into how brain networks may contribute to the experiences of psychosis, highlighting potential targets for innovative therapeutic interventions.

The impact of genetics on schizophrenia is another critical area of investigation. Family and twin studies indicate a heritable component to the disorder, suggesting that genetic predispositions may interact with environmental factors to trigger the onset of symptoms. Ongoing research is focused on identifying specific genetic markers that could help predict susceptibility to schizophrenia, paving the way for early interventions and personalised treatment approaches.

In conclusion, the intersection of neuroscience and schizophrenia research continues to evolve, providing valuable insights into the biological basis of this disorder. As our understanding deepens, it becomes increasingly clear that a multidisciplinary approach, incorporating neuroscience, psychology, and social support, is essential for effective management and treatment of schizophrenia. This holistic perspective not only enhances our comprehension of the disorder but also empowers individuals and their families in navigating the challenges associated with it.

Neuroanatomical changes (e.g., prefrontal cortex, hippocampus)

Neuroanatomical changes play a critical role in understanding schizophrenia, particularly the alterations observed in regions such as the prefrontal cortex and hippocampus. The prefrontal cortex is integral to higher cognitive functions, including decision-making, impulse control, and emotional regulation. Research has shown that individuals with schizophrenia often exhibit reduced volume and activity in this area, which may contribute to the cognitive deficits and disorganisation of thought commonly associated with the disorder.

The hippocampus, a region essential for memory formation and spatial navigation, also shows significant neuroanatomical changes in those with schizophrenia. Studies indicate that individuals may experience a decrease in hippocampal volume, which could be linked to the memory impairment and difficulties with learning that are prevalent in this population. These changes may arise from a combination of genetic, environmental, and neurodevelopmental factors, emphasising the complexity of the disorder.

Furthermore, neuroimaging studies have provided insight into the connectivity between the prefrontal cortex and hippocampus, revealing disrupted pathways that may exacerbate symptoms of schizophrenia. This disconnection could lead to challenges in integrating emotional experiences with cognitive functions, ultimately affecting daily life and social interactions. Understanding these neuroanatomical changes is essential for developing targeted treatment approaches.

The implications of these alterations extend beyond the biological; they also influence the psychosocial aspects of living with schizophrenia. Family support and therapeutic interventions can play a vital role in mitigating the effects of these neuroanatomical changes. By fostering an environment that encourages understanding and communication, families can help individuals navigate the complexities of their condition more effectively.

In conclusion, recognising the neuroanatomical changes within the prefrontal cortex and hippocampus is vital for comprehending schizophrenia. These alterations not only underline the biological underpinnings of the disorder but also highlight the importance of comprehensive treatment strategies that encompass both medical and psychosocial support. Continued research in this field promises to enhance our understanding and improve outcomes for those affected by schizophrenia.

Dopaminergic pathways (mesolimbic and mesocortical circuits)

The dopaminergic pathways, specifically the mesolimbic and mesocortical circuits, play a crucial role in the understanding of schizophrenia. These pathways are integral to the brain's reward system and are implicated in mood regulation, motivation, and cognitive functions. The mesolimbic pathway primarily connects the ventral tegmental area to the nucleus accumbens, which is associated with the modulation of emotions and the experience of pleasure. Dysregulation in this pathway is often linked to the positive symptoms of schizophrenia, such as hallucinations and delusions.

Conversely, the mesocortical pathway extends from the ventral tegmental area to the prefrontal cortex, an area responsible for higher cognitive processes, including decision-making and social behaviour. Researchers have found that impairments in this circuit can lead to negative symptoms of schizophrenia, such as social withdrawal and apathy. Understanding the distinct roles of these pathways helps in identifying the complexities of the disorder and its varied manifestations in different individuals.

Moreover, the interaction between the mesolimbic and mesocortical pathways illustrates the intricate balance required for normal brain function. An overactive mesolimbic pathway may result in excessive dopamine release, leading to psychotic symptoms, while underactivity in the mesocortical pathway can exacerbate cognitive deficits. This duality highlights the importance of targeted treatment options that can address these specific pathways to improve patient outcomes.

Recent innovations in schizophrenia research have focused on developing medications that can more precisely target these dopaminergic circuits. For instance, atypical antipsychotics aim to modulate dopamine levels in a way that alleviates symptoms without causing significant side effects. Additionally, understanding these pathways contributes to the development of psychosocial interventions that can support individuals and their families in managing the complexities of the disorder.

The stigma surrounding schizophrenia often stems from misconceptions about its causes and symptoms, many of which are linked to the dysfunction of these dopaminergic pathways. By educating the public about the biological underpinnings of the disorder, we can foster greater empathy and support for those affected. As we continue to explore the mesolimbic and mesocortical circuits, it becomes clear that a comprehensive approach, integrating both medical and social support, is essential for effective management of schizophrenia.

Glutamate and NMDA receptor dysfunction

Glutamate is a key neurotransmitter in the brain, playing a crucial role in synaptic transmission and plasticity. It is particularly important in the functioning of the NMDA (N-methyl-D-aspartate) receptors, which are vital for learning, memory, and overall cognitive function. Dysfunction in glutamate signalling and NMDA receptor activity has been implicated in various psychiatric disorders, including schizophrenia. Research suggests that abnormalities in this system may contribute to the symptoms observed in individuals with schizophrenia, such as cognitive deficits and altered perception of reality.

In schizophrenia, studies have shown that there may be an excess of glutamate in certain brain regions, leading to excitotoxicity, which can damage neurons and disrupt normal brain function. This hyperactivity of glutamate can exacerbate symptoms like hallucinations and delusions. Conversely, a deficiency in NMDA receptor function has also been linked to the negative symptoms of schizophrenia, such as social withdrawal and lack of motivation. Understanding this dual role of glutamate and NMDA receptors is essential for comprehending the complex nature of schizophrenia.

Treatment options targeting the glutamatergic system are currently being explored as potential therapeutic avenues for schizophrenia. Medications that modulate glutamate levels or enhance NMDA receptor function may offer new hope for individuals struggling with this disorder. Furthermore, the integration of family support in the management of schizophrenia can play a significant role in the effectiveness of these treatment options, as families can help monitor symptoms and encourage adherence to prescribed therapies.

In addition to pharmacological interventions, lifestyle changes and coping strategies can also aid individuals with schizophrenia. Encouraging a balanced diet, regular exercise, and cognitive behavioural therapy may help alleviate some of the symptoms associated with glutamate and NMDA receptor dysfunction. It is important for patients and their families to be educated about the nature of these dysfunctions, as well as the potential for recovery through a combination of treatments and support systems.

The stigma surrounding schizophrenia often leads to misconceptions about the disorder, preventing individuals from seeking help. By fostering a deeper understanding of the biological underpinnings of schizophrenia, including the roles of glutamate and NMDA receptors, we can challenge these myths and empower those affected by the condition. Increased awareness can promote acceptance and encourage open discussions about the challenges faced by individuals living with schizophrenia, ultimately leading to better management and support.

Role of inflammation and immune system (microglial activation)

Inflammation and the immune system play a pivotal role in the pathophysiology of schizophrenia, particularly through the activation of microglia. Microglia are the resident immune cells of the central nervous system, and they are responsible for maintaining homeostasis and responding to injury or disease. In individuals with schizophrenia, these cells can become overactive, leading to chronic inflammation that may contribute to the onset and progression of the disorder. This dysregulation can manifest in various ways, influencing both the biological and psychological dimensions of schizophrenia.

Research has indicated that elevated levels of pro-inflammatory cytokines are often found in patients diagnosed with schizophrenia. These cytokines are signalling molecules that mediate inflammation and can affect neurotransmitter systems, potentially disrupting the delicate balance of neurochemicals in the brain. Such disturbances may lead to symptoms such as hallucinations and cognitive dysfunction, which are hallmark features of the illness. Understanding the relationship between inflammation and neurotransmitter alterations is crucial in comprehending how microglial activation impacts the symptoms of schizophrenia.

Moreover, the activation of microglia may not only contribute to the symptoms of schizophrenia but could also influence the effectiveness of treatment options. Antipsychotic medications, commonly used to manage schizophrenia, might have varying degrees of efficacy based on an individual's inflammatory status. As such, a better understanding of microglial activation and its consequences could pave the way for more tailored treatment approaches, potentially improving outcomes for individuals with schizophrenia.

Family support plays a significant role in managing schizophrenia, especially when considering the immune system's involvement. Families can assist in recognising early warning signs and seeking appropriate medical intervention. Moreover, a supportive environment can help mitigate stress, which is known to exacerbate inflammation. Encouraging open communication and education about the role of inflammation in schizophrenia can empower families to be more proactive in their loved ones' treatment journey.

In conclusion, the intricate relationship between inflammation, the immune system, and microglial activation is an emerging area of interest in schizophrenia research. As we delve deeper into the biological underpinnings of the disorder, it becomes evident that addressing inflammation may not only enhance our understanding of schizophrenia but also improve therapeutic strategies. Continued exploration in this field is essential for breaking down the stigma surrounding schizophrenia and fostering a more informed public dialogue about its complexities.

Genetics and Epigenetics

Genetics and epigenetics play a significant role in understanding schizophrenia, a complex mental health condition. Genetic factors contribute to an individual's susceptibility to schizophrenia, with numerous studies indicating that individuals with a family history of the disorder are at a higher risk. The interplay of multiple genes, rather than a single gene, is believed to influence the development of schizophrenia, indicating that it is a heritable condition. This genetic predisposition does not guarantee the onset of the disorder, highlighting the importance of environmental factors in its manifestation.

Epigenetics adds another layer to our understanding of schizophrenia by examining how environmental influences can affect gene expression. Factors such as stress, trauma, and substance abuse can lead to epigenetic modifications that may trigger or exacerbate the symptoms of schizophrenia in genetically predisposed individuals. This concept underscores the dynamic interaction between genes and the environment, suggesting that while one may inherit a risk for schizophrenia, lifestyle and external factors can significantly influence whether or not the disorder develops.

Research has shown that epigenetic changes can be reversible, offering potential avenues for treatment and intervention. For instance, therapies aimed at altering epigenetic markers may provide innovative strategies to manage or even prevent the development of schizophrenia in individuals at risk. Understanding these mechanisms opens up new possibilities for personalised medicine, where treatment plans can be tailored to the individual's genetic and epigenetic profiles, potentially improving outcomes.

Furthermore, the role of family support cannot be understated in the context of genetics and epigenetics. Families with a history of schizophrenia can benefit from education about the condition, enabling them to provide better support for affected members. This supportive environment can help mitigate some of the adverse effects of environmental stressors, thereby potentially influencing epigenetic factors and reducing the risk of developing the disorder.

In conclusion, the intricate relationship between genetics, epigenetics, and schizophrenia highlights the need for a multifaceted approach to treatment and management. While genetic predispositions are critical, the influence of environmental factors and family support play pivotal roles in the disorder's development and progression. Ongoing research in this field holds promise for future innovations that could lead to effective prevention and treatment strategies for schizophrenia, addressing both its biological and psychosocial dimensions.

Risk genes (e.g., DISC1, COMT, 22q11.2 deletion)

The study of risk genes associated with schizophrenia has gained significant attention in recent years, particularly genes such as DISC1, COMT, and the 22q11.2 deletion. These genes are believed to play crucial roles in the neurobiological mechanisms underlying the disorder. DISC1, or Disrupted in Schizophrenia 1, has been linked to various brain functions, including neural development and synaptic transmission, making it a focal point for understanding how disruptions in these processes can lead to the onset of schizophrenia.

COMT, or Catechol-O-Methyltransferase, is another important gene implicated in schizophrenia. It is involved in the metabolism of dopamine, a neurotransmitter that is often dysregulated in individuals with schizophrenia. Variations in the COMT gene can affect dopamine levels, influencing both cognitive function and emotional regulation. This gene's impact on schizophrenia highlights the intricate relationship between genetics and neurotransmitter systems in the brain.

The 22q11.2 deletion syndrome is also noteworthy, as it is one of the most significant genetic risk factors for developing schizophrenia. Individuals with this deletion have a higher incidence of psychiatric disorders, including schizophrenia, compared to the general population. The presence of this deletion can disrupt multiple genes, affecting brain development and increasing vulnerability to mental health issues.

Understanding these risk genes provides valuable insight into the biological underpinnings of schizophrenia, which can inform early warning signs and treatment options. Identifying individuals who carry these genetic markers may aid in developing preventive strategies and targeted interventions, thus improving the overall management of the disorder.

Furthermore, research into risk genes not only enhances the scientific understanding of schizophrenia but also helps in addressing the stigma surrounding the illness. By illustrating that schizophrenia has a biological basis, it may foster greater empathy and support for affected individuals, their families, and the broader community, ultimately promoting a more informed and compassionate approach to mental health.

Heritability and gene-environment interaction

Heritability plays a crucial role in understanding schizophrenia, as research indicates that genetic factors significantly contribute to the likelihood of developing this complex disorder. Studies show that individuals with a family history of schizophrenia have a higher risk of experiencing similar mental health challenges. This genetic predisposition can be explained through various heritability estimates, which suggest that the risk of developing schizophrenia is influenced by multiple genes, each contributing a small effect. As such, the interplay of genetics and environment becomes a focal point in understanding not only the origins of schizophrenia but also its manifestations in different individuals.

Gene-environment interaction highlights the importance of environmental factors in conjunction with genetic predisposition. While an individual may carry genes associated with schizophrenia, environmental triggers such as stress, trauma, or substance abuse can significantly influence whether these genes express themselves. This concept emphasizes that schizophrenia is not solely determined by genetics, but rather a complex interplay of both inherited traits and environmental influences. The understanding of these interactions allows for a more nuanced approach to prevention and treatment strategies tailored to individual experiences.

In addition to genetic and environmental factors, the timing of exposure to certain environmental stressors can also impact the development of schizophrenia. For instance, early life experiences, including prenatal stress or adverse childhood events, may increase the likelihood of developing the disorder later in life. This aspect underscores the importance of early intervention and support, as addressing environmental factors during critical developmental periods could potentially mitigate the risk of schizophrenia in genetically predisposed individuals.

Family support plays a pivotal role in managing schizophrenia, particularly in the context of gene-environment interactions. Families can provide a supportive environment that may help buffer against the negative effects of environmental stressors. Moreover, understanding the hereditary nature of schizophrenia can empower families to seek early warning signs in their loved ones, facilitating timely interventions that can lead to better outcomes. Thus, the role of family is not only crucial in treatment but also in fostering resilience against potential triggers associated with the disorder.

In conclusion, the exploration of heritability and gene-environment interaction in schizophrenia highlights the complexity of this mental health condition. It is essential to recognise that both genetic and environmental factors contribute to the risk of developing schizophrenia, and addressing these elements through comprehensive support systems can significantly impact individuals' lives. By promoting awareness of these dynamics, we can challenge misconceptions surrounding schizophrenia and encourage a more informed and empathetic approach to those affected by the disorder.

Brain Imaging and Biomarkers

Brain imaging techniques have revolutionised our understanding of schizophrenia, offering insights into its neurobiological underpinnings. Advanced methods such as magnetic resonance imaging (MRI) and positron emission tomography (PET) allow researchers to visualise brain structure and function in individuals diagnosed with this complex disorder. These images reveal structural abnormalities, such as enlarged ventricles and reduced grey matter, which are often associated with the symptoms of schizophrenia. By identifying these changes, scientists can better understand the brain's role in the onset and progression of the illness.

Biomarkers are another critical area of research in schizophrenia, as they provide measurable indicators of the disease. These biological markers can be derived from brain imaging or biological samples, such as blood or cerebrospinal fluid. The goal is to find specific biomarkers that can predict the onset of schizophrenia or the likelihood of a particular treatment being effective. This could lead to personalised treatment options, allowing for a more tailored approach to managing the disorder, which is crucial given the wide variability in symptoms and responses to treatment among individuals.

Additionally, the integration of brain imaging and biomarkers could significantly enhance early warning signs of schizophrenia. By observing changes in brain activity or structure before the full onset of symptoms, healthcare providers may be able to intervene sooner, potentially altering the course of the illness. This proactive approach is particularly vital for adolescents, who may be at a higher risk of developing schizophrenia. Early detection and intervention can lead to improved outcomes and a better quality of life for those affected.

Family support plays a pivotal role in managing schizophrenia, and understanding the biological aspects through brain imaging can empower families. By educating families about the neurobiological factors contributing to their loved one's condition, they can better support treatment plans and cope with the challenges of the illness. This knowledge can also help reduce the stigma surrounding schizophrenia, as it shifts the focus from character flaws to biological realities, fostering compassion and understanding within the family unit.

Finally, the continuous advancements in brain imaging and biomarker research signify hope for the future of schizophrenia treatment. Innovations in technology are likely to yield more precise and effective strategies for managing the disorder. As researchers uncover more about the brain's complexities, the potential for new therapies and interventions increases. Ultimately, the combination of these scientific advancements and strong family support can help individuals with schizophrenia lead fulfilling lives, while also addressing the myths and misconceptions that often accompany the disorder.

MRI, PET scan findings

Magnetic Resonance Imaging (MRI) and Positron Emission Tomography (PET) scans have emerged as vital tools in understanding the neurobiological underpinnings of schizophrenia. MRI provides detailed images of the brain's structure, allowing researchers to observe abnormalities that may be associated with the disorder. These structural anomalies often include alterations in the size of certain brain regions, which can be indicative of schizophrenia's impact on brain development and function. As such, MRI findings contribute significantly to early diagnosis and understanding of the condition.

On the other hand, PET scans offer insights into the brain's metabolic activity. This imaging technique measures blood flow and the uptake of glucose, which is crucial for understanding how the brain functions in individuals with schizophrenia. Research has shown that individuals with schizophrenia often exhibit altered patterns of glucose metabolism, particularly in areas related to cognition and emotion regulation. These findings can help in identifying potential targets for treatment and interventions, ultimately improving patient outcomes.

A combination of MRI and PET findings has led to a more comprehensive understanding of schizophrenia, revealing that it is not merely a psychological disorder but one rooted in biological changes within the brain. This dual approach allows for a more nuanced perspective, acknowledging the interplay between genetic predispositions and environmental factors that can trigger the onset of symptoms. It is essential to integrate this knowledge into treatment options, ensuring that therapies are tailored to the individual's specific brain function and structure.

Moreover, the findings from these imaging techniques can also play a crucial role in addressing the stigma surrounding schizophrenia. By demonstrating that schizophrenia has identifiable biological markers, it can help to dispel myths that the disorder is purely a product of personal weakness or poor character. Educating the public on the scientific basis of schizophrenia can foster a more compassionate understanding, thereby encouraging families and communities to support those affected by the disorder.

In conclusion, the advancements in MRI and PET scan technologies have transformed the landscape of schizophrenia research and treatment. As our understanding deepens, these imaging modalities not only aid in the early detection and diagnosis but also enhance our comprehension of the disorder's complexity. This knowledge is pivotal for developing innovative treatments and coping strategies, ultimately improving the quality of life for individuals living with schizophrenia.

Functional connectivity disruptions

Functional connectivity disruptions refer to the alterations in the communication pathways between different regions of the brain. In individuals with schizophrenia, these disruptions can manifest as irregular patterns of brain activity. This phenomenon is believed to contribute to the cognitive and perceptual disturbances commonly associated with the disorder, such as hallucinations and delusions. Understanding these disruptions is crucial for developing effective treatment strategies and improving outcomes for those affected by schizophrenia.

Research has identified several key areas of the brain that show significant connectivity issues in schizophrenia patients. The prefrontal cortex, responsible for decision-making and social behaviour, often exhibits decreased connectivity with other regions. Additionally, the default mode network, which is active during rest and involved in self-referential thought, also shows abnormal connectivity patterns. These findings suggest that the brain's ability to integrate information across different areas is compromised, leading to the symptoms observed in schizophrenia.

Functional connectivity disruptions can also vary between adolescents and adults with schizophrenia. In younger individuals, the brain is still developing, which may make them more susceptible to the effects of these disruptions. Early intervention and targeted treatment options can be essential in addressing these issues before they lead to more severe cognitive impairments. This highlights the importance of recognising early warning signs and providing appropriate support to adolescents at risk of developing schizophrenia.

Family support plays a vital role in managing the effects of functional connectivity disruptions. Families can help individuals with schizophrenia navigate their challenges by providing emotional support and encouraging adherence to treatment plans. Educating family members about the disorder and its symptoms can foster a more supportive environment, which is essential for recovery. Open communication within families can also help reduce stigma and misconceptions surrounding schizophrenia, making it easier for individuals to seek help.

Innovations in schizophrenia research continue to shed light on functional connectivity disruptions and their implications for treatment. Advances in neuroimaging techniques allow researchers to observe brain activity in real-time and identify specific connectivity patterns associated with schizophrenia. This knowledge paves the way for developing new therapeutic interventions that target these disruptions, ultimately improving the quality of life for those living with the disorder and addressing the stigma that often accompanies it.

Historical Perspectives

The historical perspectives on schizophrenia provide a crucial context for understanding the complexities of this mental health condition. Throughout history, individuals exhibiting symptoms of schizophrenia were often misunderstood, leading to various societal reactions ranging from fear and ostracism to misguided attempts at treatment. Ancient civilisations attributed such behaviours to spiritual or supernatural forces, viewing those affected as possessed or cursed, which significantly influenced their treatment and care.

As the understanding of mental illness evolved, the 19th century marked a pivotal shift towards more scientific approaches. During this period, the work of pioneering figures such as Emil Kraepelin began to shape the modern diagnostic criteria for schizophrenia. Kraepelin's classification of mental disorders laid the groundwork for recognising schizophrenia as a distinct illness, differentiating it from other forms of madness, which was an essential step in reducing the stigma associated with the condition.

The 20th century witnessed further advancements in the understanding and treatment of schizophrenia, particularly with the advent of psychoanalysis and later, pharmacological treatments. The introduction of antipsychotic medications in the 1950s revolutionised the management of schizophrenia, offering relief to many who had previously been confined to asylums. This era also highlighted the importance of integrating family support and community care into treatment plans, recognising the significant role that social networks play in recovery.

Despite these advancements, myths and misconceptions surrounding schizophrenia persist, often perpetuated by media portrayals and societal stigma. Many still associate schizophrenia with violence or unpredictability, which is not reflective of the majority of individuals living with the disorder. Addressing these misconceptions through education and open dialogue is essential for fostering a more supportive environment for those affected by schizophrenia and their families.

In contemporary times, research continues to uncover the biological, psychological, and social factors that contribute to schizophrenia. Innovations in neuroscience and genetic studies are paving the way for more personalised treatment options, enhancing the hope for better management strategies. Understanding the historical context of schizophrenia not only enriches our knowledge of the disorder but also encourages a more compassionate approach towards those living with it today.

Eugen Bleuler (Swiss Psychiatrist) and schizophrenia

Eugen Bleuler was a pioneering Swiss psychiatrist who played a crucial role in the understanding of schizophrenia, a complex mental health disorder. In the early 20th century, Bleuler introduced the term "schizophrenia" to describe a range of psychological phenomena that were previously misunderstood and often mislabelled. His work was instrumental in shifting the perception of the disorder from a mere set of symptoms to a more nuanced understanding that encompasses a spectrum of experiences and behaviours. Bleuler's insights laid the groundwork for modern psychiatric practices and continue to influence the field today.

One of Bleuler's significant contributions was his emphasis on the concept of "splitting of the mind" which he believed characterised schizophrenia. This idea encompassed not only the fragmentation of thoughts and emotions but also the disconnection between a person's perception of reality and their internal experiences. Bleuler identified four fundamental symptoms of schizophrenia: affective blunting, autism, ambivalence, and associative looseness. These symptoms provided a framework for clinicians to better assess and understand the disorder, leading to more effective treatment options in subsequent years.

In Bleuler's view, the onset of schizophrenia often manifested in early adulthood, with symptoms that could vary widely among individuals. He highlighted the importance of early intervention, suggesting that recognising the initial signs could lead to more favourable outcomes. This perspective has shaped contemporary approaches to identifying early warning signs of schizophrenia, which is crucial for timely treatment and support. By understanding these early manifestations, families and healthcare professionals can collaborate effectively to provide the necessary care and resources.

Bleuler also recognised the significant impact of social and familial support in managing schizophrenia. He believed that a supportive environment could greatly influence the course of the illness, emphasising that family dynamics and social interactions play a vital role in the recovery process. His advocacy for the inclusion of family members in treatment plans has since been adopted widely, reinforcing the idea that a strong support network is essential for individuals living with schizophrenia.

Finally, Bleuler's work dispelled many myths and misconceptions surrounding schizophrenia. By promoting awareness and understanding of the disorder, he sought to reduce the stigma often associated with mental illness. His legacy continues to inspire innovations in schizophrenia research and treatment, with a focus on holistic approaches that address the complex interplay of psychological, biological, and social factors. As we advance our understanding of schizophrenia, Bleuler's contributions remind us of the importance of compassion, support, and informed care in the lives of those affected by this challenging condition.

Emil Kraepelin (German Psychiatrist) and schizophrenia

Emil Kraepelin, a prominent German psychiatrist of the late 19th and early 20th centuries, made significant contributions to our understanding of mental disorders, particularly schizophrenia. He was instrumental in classifying mental illnesses and introduced the concept of manic-depressive illness. Kraepelin believed that schizophrenia was a distinct disorder, characterised by a range of symptoms that affected thought processes, emotions, and behaviour. His pioneering work laid the foundation for modern psychiatric diagnosis and treatment approaches, emphasising the need for a systematic classification of mental health issues.

Kraepelin's observations on schizophrenia were groundbreaking for their time. He noted that the disorder often presented with episodes of psychosis, including hallucinations and delusions, which could severely impair an individual's functioning. His meticulous documentation of patient cases highlighted the variability and complexity of schizophrenia, prompting further research into its underlying causes. Kraepelin's emphasis on the biological underpinnings of mental disorders marked a shift in how psychiatry viewed conditions like schizophrenia, steering the field towards a more medical model of understanding.

In his classification system, Kraepelin distinguished between different forms of schizophrenia, recognising that the disorder could manifest in various ways. This approach not only helped clinicians identify and treat individuals more effectively but also contributed to the debunking of myths surrounding schizophrenia. By defining specific subtypes, he provided a clearer framework for understanding the nuances of the disorder, which is essential for both treatment and support. This classification remains influential in contemporary psychiatric practice, as it informs diagnosis and therapeutic strategies.

Kraepelin also advocated for the importance of family support in the management of schizophrenia. He understood that the impact of the disorder extended beyond the individual, affecting families and communities. His insights underscored the need for a holistic approach to treatment, which includes psychological support for both patients and their families. This recognition of the familial context is crucial, as it fosters a supportive environment that can enhance treatment outcomes and reduce the stigma surrounding mental illness.

Emil Kraepelin's legacy in the field of psychiatry continues to resonate today, particularly in the context of schizophrenia. His work has paved the way for ongoing research and innovations in treatment options, highlighting the importance of understanding early warning signs and co-occurring disorders. As we continue to explore the complexities of schizophrenia, Kraepelin's contributions remind us of the importance of compassion, support, and informed care in the journey towards recovery.

Sigmund Freud (Neurologist, Psychoanalyst) and schizophrenia

Sigmund Freud, the father of psychoanalysis, made significant contributions to our understanding of mental health conditions, including schizophrenia. Freud proposed that schizophrenia arises from unresolved conflicts within the psyche, particularly involving the unconscious mind. His theories emphasised the importance of early childhood experiences and the impact of these on adult mental health. This perspective opened the door for further exploration into the psychological underpinnings of schizophrenia, moving beyond the purely neurological explanations prevalent at the time.

Freud's work highlighted the complex relationship between neurology and psychology in understanding schizophrenia. He believed that symptoms such as delusions and hallucinations could be interpreted as manifestations of deeper psychological conflicts. By focusing on the interplay between the conscious and unconscious mind, Freud provided a framework for understanding how internal struggles could manifest as severe mental health issues. His emphasis on the mind's complexities challenged the notion that schizophrenia was solely a biological disorder.

Despite Freud's pioneering ideas, his theories on schizophrenia have been met with criticism. Some argue that his focus on psychosexual development and unconscious conflicts overshadows the biological and genetic factors that also play a crucial role in the condition. However, Freud's insistence on considering the individual's personal history in treatment has influenced modern therapeutic practices. Today, many therapists incorporate psychodynamic approaches alongside biological treatments, acknowledging the multifaceted nature of schizophrenia.

Freud's ideas also paved the way for discussions around the stigma associated with mental illness, particularly schizophrenia. By framing the condition as a complex interplay of psychological factors, he encouraged a more compassionate view of those affected. This perspective is essential in combating the stereotypes and misconceptions that often surround schizophrenia, helping to foster a greater understanding of the condition in society.

In conclusion, Freud's contributions to the understanding of schizophrenia remain relevant in contemporary discussions about mental health. His emphasis on the psychological aspects of the condition has encouraged a holistic approach in treatment, which recognises the importance of both mind and body. As we continue to explore innovations in schizophrenia research and treatment options, Freud's legacy serves as a reminder of the need for a balanced perspective that incorporates both psychological and neurological insights.

Carl Jung (Swiss Psychiatrist and Psychoanalyst) and and schizophrenia

Carl Jung, a prominent Swiss psychiatrist and psychoanalyst, made significant contributions to the understanding of various mental health disorders, including schizophrenia. He approached this complex condition not merely as a clinical diagnosis but as a multifaceted phenomenon that intertwines with the individual's psyche and social environment. Jung's theories proposed that schizophrenia could be viewed through a lens of archetypes and the collective unconscious, offering a unique perspective on the experiences of those affected by the disorder.

Jung was particularly interested in the symptoms of schizophrenia, such as hallucinations and delusions, which he believed could represent deeper psychological conflicts. He theorised that these manifestations were not simply pathological but could reveal unresolved issues within the individual's unconscious mind. By interpreting these symptoms, Jung aimed to help patients uncover hidden aspects of their psyche, facilitating a journey towards self-discovery and integration.

In his work, Jung also emphasised the importance of the therapeutic relationship, advocating for a supportive and understanding environment in which patients could explore their experiences. He believed that the role of the therapist was not just to treat symptoms but to engage with the individual's inner world, fostering a space for healing. This approach aligns with contemporary views on the importance of family support and community involvement in the management of schizophrenia.

Jung's insights into schizophrenia have paved the way for further research into the disorder, influencing both psychoanalytic and psychotherapeutic practices. His ideas have encouraged an exploration of the links between schizophrenia and creativity, suggesting that the experiences of individuals with this condition could contribute to artistic expression and innovation. This perspective challenges prevailing myths and misconceptions about schizophrenia, highlighting the potential for personal growth amidst mental health challenges.

Ultimately, Jung's contributions to the understanding of schizophrenia remind us of the complexity of the human mind. By recognising the interplay between psychological symptoms and personal narratives, we can foster a more compassionate and informed approach to schizophrenia. His legacy continues to inspire those who seek to understand and support individuals living with this condition, promoting a holistic view of mental health that encompasses both clinical and existential dimensions.

Eric Kandel (Nobel Prize-winning Neuroscientist) and schizophrenia

Eric Kandel, a Nobel Prize-winning neuroscientist, has made significant contributions to our understanding of the biological basis of learning and memory, which are crucial areas of research in relation to schizophrenia. His work has focused on the molecular mechanisms that underlie synaptic plasticity, the process through which connections between neurons strengthen or weaken in response to activity. This research is particularly relevant to schizophrenia, as it is believed that disruptions in these mechanisms may contribute to the cognitive deficits often observed in individuals with the disorder.

Kandel's insights into synaptic changes have opened new avenues for exploring the neurobiological underpinnings of schizophrenia. By understanding how memory and learning processes are altered in those with the disorder, researchers can begin to identify potential early warning signs. For instance, difficulties in attention and memory, which are common in schizophrenia, may be linked to the synaptic alterations Kandel has studied. This connection highlights the importance of recognising these symptoms early on, as they can be critical in initiating timely treatment.

Moreover, Kandel's research underscores the potential for innovative treatment options for schizophrenia. As we learn more about the molecular pathways involved in synaptic plasticity, it may become possible to develop targeted therapies that address the specific cognitive impairments associated with the disorder. Such advancements could revolutionise how we approach schizophrenia treatment, moving beyond traditional antipsychotic medications to more nuanced interventions that consider the underlying neurobiology.

In addition to his scientific contributions, Kandel has also been an advocate for understanding the broader implications of schizophrenia on individuals and their families. He emphasises the role of family support in managing the disorder, recognising that a supportive environment can significantly enhance the effectiveness of treatment. This perspective is vital, as it encourages families to engage actively in the recovery process, helping to dispel myths and misconceptions about schizophrenia that can lead to stigma.

Finally, Kandel's emphasis on education and awareness is crucial in combating the stigma surrounding schizophrenia. By sharing his findings and promoting a deeper understanding of the disorder, he aims to foster a more empathetic society that supports those affected. His work not only contributes to scientific knowledge but also serves as a reminder of the human side of schizophrenia, highlighting the need for compassion and support for individuals navigating the complexities of this condition.

Iain McGilchrist (Neuropsychiatrist, author of The Master and His Emissary) and schizophrenia

Iain McGilchrist, a distinguished neuropsychiatrist and author of "The Master and His Emissary," provides a profound perspective on the complexities of schizophrenia. His exploration delves into the interplay between the brain's left and right hemispheres, suggesting that schizophrenia may not merely be a disorder of thought, but rather a disruption in the balance of these hemispheric functions. McGilchrist posits that the left hemisphere tends to dominate in individuals with schizophrenia, leading to a narrowed focus on details at the expense of broader contextual understanding. This imbalance can contribute to the fragmented experiences and perceptions often reported by those living with this mental health condition.

In his work, McGilchrist highlights early warning signs of schizophrenia, advocating for a timely recognition of symptoms. He underscores the importance of awareness among family and friends, as they often play a crucial role in identifying changes in behaviour or mood that may signal the onset of this disorder. By fostering a supportive environment, loved ones can help individuals seek treatment earlier, potentially improving their outcomes. McGilchrist's insights emphasise that understanding these signs can be instrumental in the effective management of schizophrenia.

Treatment options for schizophrenia are also a significant focus within McGilchrist's discussions. He advocates for a holistic approach that considers not just medication but also psychotherapy, lifestyle changes, and social support. This multifaceted strategy aims to address the various dimensions of the disorder, recognising that effective treatment must be tailored to the individual's unique experiences and challenges. McGilchrist's emphasis on a comprehensive treatment plan echoes the growing recognition of the need for integrated care in mental health.

Moreover, McGilchrist explores the impact of schizophrenia on daily life, detailing how the disorder affects not only the individual but also their families and communities. He delves into the stigma surrounding schizophrenia, which can exacerbate feelings of isolation and misunderstanding. By addressing these societal misconceptions, McGilchrist advocates for a more compassionate and informed approach to those affected by schizophrenia, highlighting the importance of empathy and support in the recovery journey.

Finally, McGilchrist's contributions to the field extend to innovations in schizophrenia research. He encourages ongoing exploration into the neurobiological underpinnings of the disorder, as well as the development of new therapies informed by cutting-edge research. His commitment to advancing understanding in this area reflects a broader movement within psychiatry to bridge the gap between neuroscience and clinical practice ultimately aiming to improve the lives of individuals with schizophrenia and their families.

Symptoms and Types

Schizophrenia is a complex mental health condition characterised by a range of symptoms that can significantly affect an individual's perception of reality. Common symptoms include hallucinations, delusions, disorganised thinking, and impaired functioning. Hallucinations may involve hearing voices or seeing things that are not present, causing distress and confusion for the individual. Delusions refer to firmly held false beliefs that can lead to paranoia or significant misinterpretations of reality, which are often resistant to contrary evidence.

There are various types of schizophrenia, each presenting with different symptoms and characteristics. The most recognised type is paranoid schizophrenia, where individuals experience intense paranoia and auditory hallucinations. On the other hand, disorganised schizophrenia is marked by disorganised speech and behaviour, making it difficult for individuals to carry out daily tasks. Catatonic schizophrenia, though less common, involves motor behaviour that can range from extreme agitation to complete immobility, highlighting the diverse manifestations of this disorder.

Recognising the early warning signs of schizophrenia is crucial for timely intervention and treatment. Symptoms may initially appear as subtle changes in behaviour, including social withdrawal, decreased motivation, or changes in personal hygiene. These early signs can often be dismissed or attributed to stress or adolescence, particularly in younger individuals. However, awareness of these signs can help family members and friends provide necessary support and encourage those affected to seek professional help.

Treatment options for schizophrenia are varied and should be tailored to the individual's needs. A combination of medication, such as antipsychotics, and psychotherapy is often the most effective approach. Psychosocial interventions, including support groups and family therapy, play a vital role in recovery. These interventions not only help individuals manage their symptoms but also improve their quality of life by fostering a supportive environment that addresses both the individual and their family's needs.

The impact of schizophrenia on daily life can be profound, affecting relationships, employment, and overall well-being. Stigma surrounding the disorder often exacerbates these challenges, leading to isolation and discrimination. Understanding the types and symptoms of schizophrenia is essential for reducing stigma and fostering an environment of support. By educating ourselves and others, we can challenge misconceptions and promote a more compassionate approach to those living with this condition.

2

Chapter 2: Early Warning Signs of Schizophrenia

Recognising Early Symptoms

Recognising the early symptoms of schizophrenia is crucial for effective intervention and treatment. Often, the onset of this mental health condition can be subtle, making it difficult for both individuals and their families to identify. Common early signs include changes in behaviour, such as withdrawal from social interactions, a decline in academic or work performance, and an unusual preoccupation with certain thoughts or beliefs. These signs can easily be overlooked or misinterpreted, emphasising the need for awareness and understanding among those who may be affected.

In many cases, individuals may experience perceptual disturbances, such as hearing voices or seeing things that others do not. These auditory or visual hallucinations can be alarming and may lead to increased isolation or fear. Family members often play a critical role in recognising these signs, as they are usually the first to observe changes in a loved one's behaviour. Encouraging open communication and fostering a supportive environment can significantly aid in early detection and management.

Another important aspect to consider is the emotional state of the individual.

Symptoms such as anxiety, depression, or sudden mood swings may precede more pronounced symptoms of schizophrenia. Recognising these early emotional signals can prompt timely professional support. It is vital for both individuals and their families to understand that these emotional fluctuations are part of a larger picture and should not be dismissed as mere adolescence or typical behavioural changes.

Awareness of the broader context in which schizophrenia develops is also essential. Co-occurring disorders, such as substance abuse or anxiety disorders, can compound the challenges faced by individuals showing early symptoms. Recognising these complexities allows for a more comprehensive approach to treatment, where both schizophrenia and any co-occurring conditions can be addressed simultaneously, leading to better outcomes.

Finally, breaking the stigma surrounding schizophrenia is imperative in promoting early recognition of symptoms. By fostering an environment where mental health discussions are normalised, individuals may feel more comfortable seeking help. Educational initiatives aimed at dispelling myths and misconceptions about schizophrenia can empower families and communities to support those in need, ultimately leading to earlier diagnosis and a more effective treatment journey.

Behavioural Changes

Behavioural changes are often among the first indicators of schizophrenia, manifesting in various ways that can significantly impact an individual's daily life. These changes can include alterations in social interactions, a decline in self-care, and shifts in emotional responses. For those close to the individual, recognising these early warning signs is crucial, as they may signal the onset of a more severe episode. Understanding these changes can aid not only the individuals affected but also their families and support networks in responding appropriately.

Social withdrawal is a common behavioural change that may occur in individuals with schizophrenia. Friends and family may notice a marked decrease in communication or a reluctance to engage in previously enjoyed activities. This withdrawal can stem from a combination of symptoms such as paranoia, anxiety, or the overwhelming nature of social stimuli. It is essential to create an environment that encourages open communication, allowing individuals to express their feelings without fear of judgement or stigma.

Another significant change is the alteration in daily routines and self-care practices. Individuals may neglect personal hygiene, miss appointments, or exhibit erratic sleeping patterns. This neglect can be a result of cognitive impairments associated with schizophrenia, making it challenging for them to maintain a structured routine. Family members can play a vital role by offering support and encouraging healthy habits, which can mitigate some of these behavioural changes and enhance overall wellbeing.

Emotional responses may also become less stable, with individuals displaying inappropriate or exaggerated reactions to situations. Such changes can lead to misunderstandings and strained relationships with family and friends. Education about the condition is essential to foster empathy and patience among loved ones, helping them to better understand the emotional struggles faced by those with schizophrenia. This understanding can significantly improve the support network, leading to more effective coping strategies for everyone involved.

In conclusion, recognising and understanding behavioural changes in schizophrenia is paramount for effective management and support. These changes can profoundly affect an individual's quality of life and their relationships with others. By fostering awareness and compassion, families and friends can create a supportive environment that encourages individuals to seek treatment and engage in meaningful interactions, ultimately improving their overall experience with schizophrenia.

Importance of Early Intervention

Early intervention in schizophrenia is crucial for improving outcomes and enhancing quality of life for individuals affected by the disorder. Recognising early warning signs, such as social withdrawal, changes in mood, or unusual thoughts, allows for timely treatment and support. When intervention occurs at an early stage, it can significantly reduce the severity of symptoms and the impact on daily functioning, ultimately leading to a more favourable prognosis.

The benefits of early intervention extend beyond symptom management; it also plays a vital role in preventing the development of co-occurring disorders. Individuals with schizophrenia often face challenges related to substance abuse, depression, or anxiety. Early identification and treatment can address these issues concurrently, which is essential for comprehensive care. By tackling these co-occurring conditions alongside schizophrenia, individuals are more likely to achieve better overall mental health outcomes.

Family support is another critical aspect of early intervention. Families who are educated about the signs of schizophrenia and the importance of seeking help can act as vital advocates for their loved ones. Encouraging open communication and providing emotional support can foster a sense of stability during a turbulent time. Moreover, involving families in the treatment process can enhance the effectiveness of interventions, making it easier for individuals to adhere to their treatment plans.

Innovations in schizophrenia research have also highlighted the importance of early intervention. Studies have shown that neurobiological changes occur in the brain long before the onset of psychotic symptoms. This knowledge paves the way for preventative strategies, including education about risk factors and the implementation of screening tools. The goal is to identify individuals at risk and provide them with the necessary resources and support before the onset of more severe symptoms.

In conclusion, the importance of early intervention in schizophrenia cannot be understated. It not only facilitates better management of symptoms but also promotes overall wellbeing by addressing co-occurring disorders and involving family support. As society continues to challenge the stigma surrounding mental health, it is essential to advocate for early recognition and intervention as a standard practice. This proactive approach has the potential to transform lives and foster a greater understanding of schizophrenia as a manageable condition.

3

Chapter 3: Treatment Options for Schizophrenia

Medication Approaches

Medication approaches play a pivotal role in the management of schizophrenia, addressing both the positive and negative symptoms of the disorder. Antipsychotic medications are commonly prescribed and can significantly improve the quality of life for many individuals. These medications work by altering the levels of neurotransmitters in the brain, particularly dopamine, which has been linked to the symptoms of schizophrenia. It is essential for patients to work closely with their healthcare providers to find the most effective medication and dosage tailored to their specific needs.

In addition to traditional antipsychotics, newer atypical antipsychotics have emerged, offering different mechanisms of action and potentially fewer side effects. These medications can be particularly beneficial for individuals who may not respond well to older treatments. However, it is crucial to monitor any side effects closely, as these can impact adherence to the treatment plan. Regular consultations with healthcare professionals can help manage these side effects, ensuring that the treatment remains both effective and tolerable.

Medication alone is often not sufficient for comprehensive schizophrenia treatment. A multifaceted approach that includes psychotherapy, social support, and family involvement is vital for optimal outcomes. Cognitive-behavioural therapy (CBT) can be especially helpful in conjunction with medication, addressing the cognitive distortions and irrational fears that may arise in individuals with schizophrenia. Family support can also play a significant role, providing essential encouragement and understanding throughout the treatment process.

Despite the benefits of medication, myths and misconceptions surrounding schizophrenia can hinder treatment effectiveness. Some individuals may fear the stigma associated with the disorder, which can deter them from seeking necessary help. Education and awareness are crucial in dispelling these myths, promoting a more supportive environment for those affected. It is important for families and communities to understand that schizophrenia is a medical condition requiring appropriate treatment and support, rather than a personal failing.

In conclusion, medication approaches are a cornerstone of schizophrenia management, but they should be viewed as part of a broader treatment strategy. Combining medication with therapy and social support can lead to improved outcomes, helping individuals manage their symptoms and lead fulfilling lives. Continuous research into innovative treatment options will further enhance our understanding of schizophrenia and improve the lives of those affected. As we move forward, fostering a culture of support and understanding remains essential in combating the stigma associated with this complex disorder.

Psychotherapy and Supportive Therapies

Psychotherapy and supportive therapies play a crucial role in the comprehensive treatment of schizophrenia. These approaches provide individuals with the tools they need to cope with their symptoms and improve their overall quality of life. Psychotherapy, particularly cognitive-behavioural therapy (CBT), helps patients to identify and challenge distorted thought patterns and beliefs that can exacerbate their condition. By fostering better understanding and management of their illness, individuals are empowered to take control of their treatment process.

Supportive therapies, such as group therapy and family therapy, also contribute significantly to the recovery journey. These modalities create an environment where individuals can share their experiences and feelings with others who understand their struggles. Group therapy offers a sense of community and belonging, which can counteract the isolation often felt by those with schizophrenia. Family therapy encourages open communication among family members, helping them to understand the illness and support their loved ones more effectively.

In addition to traditional psychotherapy, innovative therapeutic approaches are emerging to enhance the treatment landscape for schizophrenia. Mindfulness-based interventions and art therapy have shown promising results in helping individuals manage stress and express their emotions. These therapies can be particularly beneficial for those who may struggle with verbal communication, providing alternative avenues for self-expression and reflection.

The integration of psychotherapy and supportive therapies into a treatment plan can also significantly reduce stigma surrounding schizophrenia. By normalising discussions about mental health and providing education to both patients and their families, these therapies foster an environment of understanding and acceptance. This shift not only benefits those directly affected by schizophrenia but also influences the broader societal perceptions of mental health disorders.

Ultimately, psychotherapy and supportive therapies are vital components of schizophrenia management. They provide individuals with essential coping strategies, foster supportive relationships, and contribute to the overall effectiveness of treatment. As research continues to evolve in this field the integration of various therapeutic approaches will likely lead to more personalised and effective care, enhancing the lives of those living with schizophrenia.

Holistic and Alternative Treatments

Holistic and alternative treatments for schizophrenia offer individuals a broader spectrum of therapeutic options that complement traditional medical approaches. These methods focus on the whole person, addressing physical, emotional, and spiritual well-being. By integrating these therapies, individuals may find enhanced relief from symptoms and improved overall quality of life. The growing interest in holistic practices reflects a desire for more personalised care and the recognition of the limitations of conventional treatments alone.

One popular alternative treatment is mindfulness and meditation, which can help reduce stress and anxiety. Practising mindfulness encourages individuals to stay present, promoting awareness of thoughts and feelings without judgment. This practice can be particularly beneficial for those experiencing early warning signs of schizophrenia, as it may assist in managing symptoms and preventing their escalation. Many individuals report feeling more centred and calm after incorporating mindfulness into their daily routines.

Nutritional therapies are another essential aspect of holistic treatments. A balanced diet rich in omega-3 fatty acids, antioxidants, and vitamins can play a crucial role in brain health. Some studies suggest that certain dietary changes may positively influence mood and cognitive function, potentially aiding in the management of schizophrenia symptoms. Consulting with a nutritionist can provide tailored dietary recommendations that support mental health alongside conventional treatments.

Family support is also vital in holistic approaches to managing schizophrenia. Engaging family members in the treatment process fosters a supportive environment that can enhance the effectiveness of various therapies. Family involvement can help address misconceptions surrounding the disorder, reduce stigma, and create a more understanding atmosphere. Open communication and education about the nature of schizophrenia can empower families to provide the necessary support for their loved ones.

In conclusion, while holistic and alternative treatments may not replace traditional medical interventions, they can serve as valuable complements.

By exploring these options, individuals with schizophrenia and their families can develop a more comprehensive management plan. This integrative approach acknowledges the complexity of the disorder and respects the unique experiences of each individual, ultimately promoting better outcomes and improved quality of life.

4

Chapter 4: Schizophrenia and Co-occurring Disorders

Common Co-occurring Conditions

Co-occurring conditions frequently accompany schizophrenia, complicating diagnosis and treatment for individuals affected by this mental health disorder. These conditions may include mood disorders, anxiety disorders, and substance use disorders, all of which can exacerbate the symptoms of schizophrenia. Understanding these co-occurring conditions is essential for effective management and care, as they can significantly affect the overall well-being and recovery process of individuals.

Mood disorders, such as depression and bipolar disorder, are particularly common among those with schizophrenia. The presence of a mood disorder can intensify feelings of hopelessness or despair, making it difficult for individuals to engage in treatment or manage their symptoms effectively. It is vital for healthcare providers to assess for these mood disorders when diagnosing and treating schizophrenia, as integrated treatment plans can lead to better outcomes.

Anxiety disorders are another prevalent issue for individuals with schizophrenia. Symptoms of anxiety can manifest as excessive worry, panic attacks, or social anxiety, which may lead to further isolation and distress. Addressing anxiety through appropriate therapeutic approaches, such as cognitive-behavioural therapy or medication, can help improve an individual's quality of life and enhance their ability to cope with the challenges presented by schizophrenia.

Substance use disorders are also commonly seen in individuals with schizophrenia, often as a means of self-medication. The use of alcohol or drugs can lead to a cycle of worsening symptoms and increased difficulty in adhering to treatment plans. Identifying and addressing substance use is crucial for effective management, as it can significantly hinder the recovery trajectory and overall mental health of those affected.

In conclusion, recognising and addressing common co-occurring conditions in individuals with schizophrenia is essential for comprehensive treatment. By understanding the interplay between schizophrenia and these additional disorders, healthcare providers can create more effective and tailored treatment plans. This holistic approach not only aids in symptom management but also promotes a better quality of life for individuals navigating the complexities of schizophrenia and its associated conditions.

Impact on Treatment and Management

The impact of schizophrenia on treatment and management cannot be overstated, as it shapes not only clinical approaches but also the overall support system surrounding individuals diagnosed with the disorder. Understanding the complexities of schizophrenia is crucial for healthcare professionals, families, and the individuals themselves. Effective management requires a combination of medication, therapy, and support, all tailored to the unique needs of the person affected. Early intervention is key, as it can significantly improve outcomes and enhance the quality of life for those living with schizophrenia.

Treatment options for schizophrenia have evolved considerably over the years, with advancements in medication leading to better symptom management and fewer side effects. Antipsychotic drugs play a pivotal role in stabilising mood and reducing the severity of psychotic symptoms. However, medication alone is often insufficient; comprehensive treatment plans that incorporate psychotherapy, psychoeducation, and social skills training are essential. These approaches not only address the symptoms but also empower individuals to manage their condition more effectively.

The role of family support in managing schizophrenia cannot be overlooked, as families often serve as the primary caregivers and advocates for their loved ones. Education about the disorder is vital for families to understand the challenges and nuances of schizophrenia, enabling them to provide informed support. By fostering a nurturing environment and open communication, families can help mitigate the stigma surrounding the illness and create a more conducive atmosphere for recovery.

Moreover, the impact of schizophrenia extends beyond the individual, affecting their daily lives and relationships. Co-occurring disorders, such as depression or substance abuse, can complicate treatment and require integrated management strategies. It is essential for treatment plans to account for these complexities, ensuring that all aspects of an individual's health are addressed. This holistic approach is vital for promoting recovery and improving overall well-being.

Innovations in schizophrenia research continue to offer hope for more effective treatment and management strategies. Ongoing studies aim to unravel the biological underpinnings of the disorder and explore novel therapeutic avenues. As our understanding of schizophrenia deepens, the potential for improved outcomes grows, highlighting the importance of continued research and collaboration among healthcare providers, researchers, and families. With the right support and intervention, individuals with schizophrenia can lead fulfilling lives, challenging the misconceptions and stigma often associated with the disorder.

Integrated Treatment Strategies

Integrated treatment strategies for schizophrenia focus on a comprehensive approach that encompasses various facets of care. This method acknowledges the complexity of the disorder, recognising that effective management often requires more than just medication. By combining pharmacological treatments with psychosocial interventions, healthcare providers can create a more supportive environment for individuals living with schizophrenia.

One of the key elements of integrated treatment is the collaboration between different healthcare professionals. Psychiatrists, psychologists, social workers, and occupational therapists often work as a cohesive team to develop tailored treatment plans. This collaborative framework ensures that all aspects of a patient's health, including mental, emotional, and social needs, are addressed comprehensively.

Family involvement plays a crucial role in the success of integrated treatment strategies. Educating family members about the disorder can significantly enhance support systems and reduce feelings of isolation for the individual. Family therapy sessions can also provide a space for open communication, helping to reduce stigma and misunderstandings related to schizophrenia.

Moreover, integrated treatment strategies often include addressing co-occurring disorders, such as substance abuse or anxiety. Recognising and treating these conditions concurrently can lead to better overall outcomes, as untreated co-occurring issues can complicate the management of schizophrenia. This holistic approach not only improves the quality of life for individuals but also fosters a sense of empowerment and agency in their treatment journey.

Finally, ongoing research into innovative treatment methods continues to shape integrated strategies. Advancements in technology and therapeutic techniques are paving the way for new interventions that can further enhance treatment efficacy. By remaining adaptable and informed about the latest findings, healthcare providers can ensure that individuals with schizophrenia receive the most effective and compassionate care possible.

5

Chapter 5: The Role of Family Support in Schizophrenia Management

Importance of Family Involvement

Family involvement plays a crucial role in the management and understanding of schizophrenia. Families often serve as the first line of support, recognising early warning signs and providing essential emotional and practical assistance. By being engaged, family members can help individuals navigate the complexities of their condition, making it easier for them to seek treatment and adhere to prescribed therapies. This involvement not only aids in symptom management but also fosters a sense of belonging and understanding that is vital for recovery.

Moreover, family support can significantly impact the overall treatment outcomes for individuals with schizophrenia. Studies have shown that when families participate in treatment planning and decision-making, patients are more likely to adhere to their treatment regimens. This collaboration can enhance communication between the patient and healthcare providers, leading to more personalised care. In essence, family members become advocates for their loved ones, ensuring that their needs and preferences are taken into account in the therapeutic process.

Understanding the nuances of schizophrenia is also easier when families are involved. They can educate themselves about the disorder, dispelling myths and misconceptions that often surround schizophrenia. This knowledge empowers families to provide informed support, reducing stigma and fostering a more supportive environment for the individual. By breaking down barriers of misunderstanding, families can create a nurturing atmosphere that encourages open dialogue and emotional expression.

In addition to practical support, family involvement can address the emotional aspects of living with schizophrenia. Individuals often experience feelings of isolation and distress; however, with the backing of their families, they are more likely to feel valued and understood. Family members can help their loved ones develop coping strategies and navigate the challenges associated with the condition. This emotional support is fundamental in helping individuals regain confidence and improve their quality of life.

Ultimately, the importance of family involvement in schizophrenia management cannot be overstated. It cultivates resilience and hope, essential components in the journey towards recovery. By fostering strong family connections, individuals can feel less alone in their struggles, leading to more positive outcomes. Therefore, encouraging family participation should be an integral part of any treatment plan for those affected by schizophrenia, highlighting the profound impact of love and support in the healing process.

Effective Communication Strategies

Effective communication is critical in managing schizophrenia, both for individuals experiencing the condition and their families. Clear and open dialogue can help in understanding the symptoms, treatment options, and the daily challenges faced by those suffering from schizophrenia. It is essential for caregivers and family members to engage in conversations that foster trust and support, as this can significantly impact the recovery process. By utilising straightforward language and avoiding assumptions, effective communication can bridge the gap between patients and their supporters.

One key strategy in effective communication is active listening. This involves giving full attention to the individual speaking, acknowledging their feelings, and validating their experiences. For individuals with schizophrenia, who may struggle with expressing their thoughts, it is vital that listeners remain patient and non-judgmental. Active listening can provide a safe space for patients to share their thoughts and concerns, which is crucial for their emotional well-being and for identifying early warning signs of relapse.

Another important aspect of communication is the use of clear and concise language. Individuals with schizophrenia may have difficulty processing complex information, making it essential to convey messages simply and directly. Avoiding jargon and technical terms can help ensure that the individual comprehends what is being discussed. Moreover, employing visual aids or written materials can enhance understanding, particularly when discussing treatment options or coping strategies.

Non-verbal communication also plays a significant role in interactions with individuals diagnosed with schizophrenia. Body language, facial expressions, and tone of voice can convey empathy and understanding, which are vital in building rapport. Being aware of one's own non-verbal cues can help prevent misunderstandings and promote a more supportive environment. Additionally, encouraging open dialogue about feelings and thoughts can empower individuals to express themselves and feel more understood.

Finally, the role of education cannot be overstated in effective communication strategies. Providing information on schizophrenia—its myths, misconceptions, and co-occurring disorders—can equip both the individual and their family with the knowledge necessary to navigate challenges. Educational resources can promote a better understanding of the condition, reduce stigma, and encourage a proactive approach to management, ultimately fostering a more supportive atmosphere for recovery.

Support Resources for Families

Families play a crucial role in the management of schizophrenia, often serving as the primary support system for individuals affected by this condition. Understanding the complexities of schizophrenia can empower families to provide better care and support. It is essential for family members to educate themselves about the disorder, including its symptoms, treatment options, and the challenges that may arise. This knowledge not only helps in recognising early warning signs but also in understanding the impact of schizophrenia on daily life and relationships.

Support resources for families are varied and can significantly enhance the coping strategies available to them. Organisations dedicated to mental health often provide educational materials, workshops, and support groups. These resources can offer a platform for families to share their experiences and learn from one another. Connecting with others facing similar challenges can alleviate feelings of isolation and provide practical advice on managing the day-to-day realities of living with someone who has schizophrenia.

In addition to peer support, professional resources are available to families. Mental health professionals can offer guidance tailored to the unique dynamics of each family. Therapists and counsellors can help family members navigate their feelings, improve communication, and develop effective strategies to support their loved one. Engaging with professionals can also facilitate a deeper understanding of co-occurring disorders that may accompany schizophrenia, further informing the family's approach to care.

Furthermore, advocacy groups play a vital role in supporting families of individuals with schizophrenia. These organisations often work to raise awareness and combat the stigma surrounding mental health issues. By participating in advocacy efforts, families can contribute to a broader societal understanding of schizophrenia, which may lead to increased resources and better treatment options in the community. This communal effort not only supports families but also fosters a more informed public perception of schizophrenia.

Lastly, it is important for families to prioritise their own mental health and well-being while supporting their loved ones. Engaging in self-care practices, seeking professional help when needed, and maintaining social connections can enhance resilience. Families must remember that they are not alone in this journey and that utilising available support resources can make a significant difference in their lives and the lives of individuals living with schizophrenia.

6

Chapter 6: Schizophrenia Myths and Misconceptions

Common Misconceptions

Many people hold misconceptions about schizophrenia that can lead to misunderstanding and stigma. One common myth is that individuals with schizophrenia have a split personality or are simply 'mad'. This conflation of schizophrenia with dissociative identity disorder (formerly known as multiple personality disorder) is not accurate. Schizophrenia affects how a person thinks, feels, and behaves, but it does not involve having multiple distinct identities. Understanding this distinction is crucial in fostering empathy and support for those affected.

Another prevalent misconception is that schizophrenia is synonymous with violence. While some media portrayals suggest that individuals with schizophrenia are dangerous, research shows that they are more likely to be victims of violence rather than perpetrators. The stigma surrounding these misconceptions can prevent individuals from seeking help and support, further isolating them in their struggles. By challenging these stereotypes, society can create a more compassionate environment for those with the condition.

Furthermore, many believe that schizophrenia is a rare disorder, when in fact, it affects approximately 1 in 100 people worldwide. This misunderstanding can lead to the underestimation of resources needed for research, treatment, and support systems. Increasing awareness of the prevalence of schizophrenia is essential in promoting better understanding and allocation of resources for those affected and their families.

Additionally, there is a belief that schizophrenia only occurs in adults, ignoring the fact that it can manifest in adolescence. Early signs can often go unnoticed or be misinterpreted as typical teenage behaviour, delaying intervention. Recognising early warning signs and understanding that schizophrenia can affect younger individuals is critical for timely treatment and support, which can significantly improve outcomes.

Lastly, misconceptions about treatment options can lead to despair among those diagnosed with schizophrenia. Some people believe that there is no effective treatment available, which is far from the truth. Advances in research have led to various treatment modalities, including medication and psychotherapy, that can help manage symptoms effectively. It is important to communicate that recovery is possible, and that individuals with schizophrenia can lead fulfilling lives with appropriate support and treatment.

The Reality of Schizophrenia

Schizophrenia is a complex and often misunderstood mental health condition that affects how individuals think, feel, and behave. Many people associate schizophrenia with severe symptoms such as hallucinations and delusions, but the reality is far more nuanced. The onset of schizophrenia typically occurs in late adolescence or early adulthood, and its symptoms can vary widely from person to person. Understanding these variations is crucial for recognising early warning signs and promoting timely intervention.

One of the most challenging aspects of schizophrenia is the stigma surrounding it. Many individuals with schizophrenia face discrimination and misunderstanding from society, which can exacerbate their condition and hinder their recovery. This stigma often stems from myths and misconceptions that portray those with schizophrenia as dangerous or incapable of leading normal lives. By educating the public and fostering a more compassionate understanding, we can help to reduce this stigma and support those affected by the disorder.

Treatment options for schizophrenia have evolved significantly over the years. While antipsychotic medications remain a cornerstone of treatment, there are now various therapeutic approaches available, including cognitive behavioural therapy and family support interventions. These treatments aim not only to alleviate symptoms but also to improve overall quality of life. The role of family support in managing schizophrenia cannot be overstated; a supportive network can provide essential emotional and practical assistance to individuals navigating their journey with the disorder.

Schizophrenia is often accompanied by co-occurring disorders, such as anxiety or substance use disorders. These comorbid conditions can complicate diagnosis and treatment, necessitating a comprehensive approach that addresses all aspects of an individual's mental health. Innovations in schizophrenia research continue to shed light on the biological and environmental factors contributing to its development, paving the way for more effective interventions and support strategies.

In conclusion, living with schizophrenia presents unique challenges that affect daily life and interpersonal relationships. However, with the right treatment and support, individuals can manage their symptoms and lead fulfilling lives. It is imperative for society as a whole to foster an environment of understanding and acceptance, breaking down the barriers of stigma and misinformation surrounding schizophrenia. Through education and advocacy, we can create a more inclusive world for those impacted by this condition.

Educating Others

Educating others about schizophrenia is crucial in dispelling myths and misconceptions that often surround this mental health condition. Many people hold inaccurate beliefs about schizophrenia, viewing it as synonymous with violence or unpredictability. By providing accurate information, we can foster a deeper understanding of the disorder, its symptoms, and what individuals living with it experience. Education serves as a powerful tool to combat stigma and promote empathy within communities.

One effective way to educate others is through community workshops and seminars. These events can provide a platform for mental health professionals, individuals with lived experience, and families affected by schizophrenia to share insights and personal stories. Such interactions not only inform attendees about early warning signs and treatment options but also encourage open discussions about the challenges faced by those with schizophrenia. Engaging the community in this way helps to create a supportive environment for individuals and families alike.

In addition to formal events, social media and online platforms offer an accessible means of sharing information about schizophrenia. By utilising these platforms, advocates can reach a broader audience and address common myths directly. Creating informative content, such as articles, videos, and infographics, can be an effective strategy to raise awareness and educate people about the realities of living with schizophrenia. This digital approach allows for continuous engagement and the ability to respond to questions or concerns in real-time.

Family support plays a vital role in the management of schizophrenia, and educating family members is equally important. Family members who understand the condition can better support their loved ones, assist in recognising early warning signs, and encourage adherence to treatment plans. Educational programmes tailored for families can help them navigate the complexities of schizophrenia, fostering resilience and understanding within the family unit.

Ultimately, educating others about schizophrenia is a collective responsibility that can lead to a more informed and compassionate society. By empowering individuals with knowledge, we can break down stigma, support those affected by schizophrenia, and ensure that they receive the understanding and care they deserve. It is through education that we can build communities that are more accepting and supportive of mental health challenges, paving the way for innovative research and effective coping strategies for individuals facing this disorder.

7

Chapter 7: Impact of Schizophrenia on Daily Life

Challenges in Daily Functioning

Living with schizophrenia presents numerous challenges that can significantly affect daily functioning. Individuals may struggle with basic tasks such as maintaining personal hygiene, adhering to medication schedules, or managing daily responsibilities like work or education. This can lead to a cycle of frustration and withdrawal, exacerbating feelings of isolation and anxiety. The impact of these challenges is not only felt by the individual but can also ripple out to affect family members and friends, who may feel helpless in supporting their loved one.

Cognitive difficulties are a common symptom of schizophrenia that can hinder daily functioning. Problems with attention, memory, and executive functioning can make it difficult for individuals to focus on tasks or organise their thoughts. This can manifest in various ways, such as forgetting appointments, struggling to follow conversations, or becoming easily overwhelmed by complex situations. These cognitive impairments often contribute to the stigma surrounding schizophrenia, as they may be misinterpreted as laziness or lack of motivation.

Social interactions can also be profoundly affected by schizophrenia. Individuals may experience paranoia or delusions that make it challenging to engage with others, leading to social withdrawal. This isolation can further deteriorate mental health, creating a vicious cycle. Family support plays a crucial role in helping individuals navigate these social challenges, as understanding and compassionate relationships can provide a buffer against the negative effects of isolation.

Moreover, the management of co-occurring disorders, such as depression or anxiety, can complicate daily functioning for those with schizophrenia. These additional mental health issues may require different treatment approaches and can exacerbate the challenges already faced. It is essential for treatment plans to address both schizophrenia and any co-occurring conditions to improve overall quality of life and functioning.

Lastly, addressing the stigma surrounding schizophrenia is vital for enhancing daily functioning. Misconceptions about the disorder often lead to discrimination, further isolating individuals and complicating their ability to seek help. Increasing public awareness and understanding can foster a more supportive environment, encouraging those affected to engage in community activities and seek the assistance they need. This societal shift is crucial for improving the daily lives of individuals living with schizophrenia.

Social Relationships and Community Integration

Social relationships and community integration play a crucial role in the lives of individuals affected by schizophrenia. The nature of these relationships can greatly influence an individual's mental health and overall well-being. Supportive friendships and community ties can help mitigate feelings of isolation and loneliness often experienced by those with the condition. Conversely, a lack of social support can exacerbate symptoms and hinder recovery, making it essential for families, friends, and community members to foster an inclusive environment.

Family support is particularly significant in the management of schizophrenia. Families can provide emotional stability and practical assistance, which are vital for individuals dealing with the challenges of the disorder. Encouraging open communication within the family can also help demystify the experience of schizophrenia, allowing family members to understand better the struggles faced by their loved ones. This understanding can lead to a more compassionate and supportive home environment, essential for recovery and management.

Community integration initiatives are equally important, as they help individuals with schizophrenia to participate actively in societal activities. Programmes that encourage social skills training and peer support can empower individuals, helping them to build meaningful connections and engage in community life. Such initiatives can reduce stigma and promote acceptance, creating a more supportive atmosphere for those living with the disorder. The more engaged individuals are within their communities, the more likely they are to experience improved mental health outcomes.

However, the stigma surrounding schizophrenia remains a significant barrier to community integration. Misconceptions about the disorder can lead to discrimination and social exclusion, further isolating those affected. It is crucial to address these myths through education and awareness campaigns that highlight the realities of living with schizophrenia. Promoting understanding can help dismantle the negative perceptions surrounding the disorder, paving the way for greater acceptance and inclusion.

In conclusion, fostering social relationships and community integration is vital for individuals with schizophrenia. By encouraging supportive family dynamics and community involvement, we can help individuals navigate their challenges more effectively. Addressing stigma and misconceptions is equally important in creating an environment conducive to recovery. Together, these elements form a comprehensive approach to improving the lives of those affected by schizophrenia, enhancing their social networks and overall quality of life.

Employment and Education Considerations

Employment and education are critical elements that can significantly impact the lives of individuals with schizophrenia. Many people diagnosed with this condition face challenges in maintaining stable employment and pursuing educational opportunities due to the nature of their symptoms. Early intervention and appropriate support can help individuals navigate these challenges, enabling them to achieve greater independence and a sense of purpose. Employers and educational institutions play a vital role in fostering environments that are inclusive and supportive of individuals with mental health conditions.

One of the primary considerations for individuals with schizophrenia is the need for flexible employment options. Many find traditional work environments overwhelming, leading to increased stress and potential exacerbation of symptoms. Job accommodations, such as flexible hours or remote work opportunities, can be beneficial. Furthermore, vocational training programmes tailored for those with mental health issues can help individuals build skills and confidence, ultimately enhancing their employability and job satisfaction.

Education also plays a significant role in the lives of those with schizophrenia. Many individuals may experience disruptions in their academic pursuits due to their condition. Supportive educational settings that understand the unique needs of these individuals can make a substantial difference. This includes access to mental health resources on campus, as well as academic accommodations that allow for a more manageable workload, enabling students to thrive academically without compromising their well-being.

Family support is another crucial factor in navigating employment and education for individuals with schizophrenia. Families can provide encouragement and practical assistance, helping to create a stable foundation for their loved ones. Open communication about the challenges faced can lead to better understanding and commitment to support systems that foster both educational and occupational success. Moreover, families can advocate for their loved ones, ensuring they receive the necessary resources and support from educational institutions and employers.

Finally, addressing the stigma surrounding schizophrenia is essential for improving employment and education outcomes. Misconceptions and negative stereotypes can hinder opportunities for individuals, making it imperative for society to foster a more accepting environment. Educational programmes aimed at raising awareness about schizophrenia can help dismantle these myths, encouraging a culture of inclusivity and understanding. By promoting acceptance and support, we can enhance the quality of life for those living with schizophrenia, empowering them to pursue their aspirations in both education and employment.

8

Chapter 8: Schizophrenia in Adolescents vs. Adults

Differences in Onset and Symptoms

The onset of schizophrenia can vary significantly between individuals, often presenting itself in different ways and at different stages of life. For some, symptoms may emerge gradually over months or years, while others may experience a sudden onset of psychotic symptoms. This variability can make early identification challenging, as the initial signs may be subtle and easily overlooked. Understanding these differences in onset is crucial for timely intervention and treatment, which can greatly influence the course of the disorder.

Symptoms of schizophrenia also differ widely among individuals, encompassing a range of cognitive, emotional, and behavioural aspects. Positive symptoms, such as hallucinations and delusions, are often the most recognised, but negative symptoms like apathy, social withdrawal, and lack of motivation can be equally debilitating. Additionally, cognitive symptoms affecting memory and attention may also emerge, complicating the overall picture of the disorder. A comprehensive understanding of these symptoms is essential for effective diagnosis and management.

In adolescents, the onset of schizophrenia often coincides with significant developmental changes, which can further complicate recognition and treatment. Symptoms may be mistaken for typical teenage behaviour, leading to delays in diagnosis and support. Conversely, adults may present with a different symptom profile, often reflecting their life experiences and coping strategies. Recognising these age-related differences can help families and healthcare providers tailor treatment approaches to meet the specific needs of individuals at different life stages.

Co-occurring disorders, such as depression or substance abuse, can also influence the onset and manifestation of schizophrenia symptoms. These comorbid conditions can exacerbate the primary disorder, leading to a more complex clinical picture and necessitating integrated treatment strategies. Understanding how these disorders interact is vital for developing effective management plans that address all aspects of an individual's mental health.

Finally, the role of family support cannot be overstated in managing schizophrenia. Families often play a critical role in recognising early warning signs and advocating for appropriate care. By fostering a supportive environment, families can help individuals navigate the challenges of the disorder, promoting adherence to treatment and improving overall quality of life. Awareness of the differences in onset and symptoms is essential not only for healthcare professionals but also for families and individuals affected by schizophrenia, as it lays the groundwork for understanding and navigating this complex condition.

Treatment Approaches for Different Age Groups

Treatment approaches for schizophrenia must be tailored to the specific age group of the individual, as developmental stages significantly influence the manifestation and management of the disorder. Children and adolescents often exhibit different symptoms compared to adults, necessitating early intervention strategies that focus on education, therapy, and family involvement. For younger patients, establishing a supportive environment and integrating treatment into their daily routines can enhance their overall well-being and recovery prospects.

In adults, treatment typically involves a combination of pharmacological interventions and psychotherapy. Antipsychotic medications play a crucial role in managing symptoms, while cognitive behavioural therapy (CBT) can help individuals develop coping strategies and address the misconceptions surrounding their condition. Support groups and community resources further aid in creating a holistic approach to treatment, fostering a sense of belonging and reducing the stigma often associated with schizophrenia.

Older adults may experience unique challenges related to schizophrenia, including comorbidities and cognitive decline. Treatment strategies for this demographic often require adjustments to medication and increased focus on psychosocial support. Engaging family members in the treatment process can also prove beneficial, as they can help monitor changes in behaviour and provide emotional support during challenging times.

Innovations in schizophrenia research have led to the development of new treatment modalities that cater to the needs of various age groups. For instance, ongoing studies are exploring the efficacy of digital therapeutics and telepsychiatry, which can enhance accessibility for individuals who may have difficulty attending traditional therapy sessions. These advancements have the potential to revolutionise treatment, making it more adaptable and responsive to individual needs.

Ultimately, the role of family support remains paramount across all age groups affected by schizophrenia. Families can provide a critical safety net, offering encouragement and understanding that can significantly influence treatment outcomes. By fostering open communication and actively participating in the management of the disorder, families can help dismantle the stigma and misconceptions surrounding schizophrenia, creating a more supportive environment for recovery.

Long-term Outcomes

Long-term outcomes for individuals diagnosed with schizophrenia can vary significantly, influenced by a myriad of factors including the severity of the disorder, the age of onset, and the availability of treatment options. Research indicates that while some individuals may experience a reduction in symptoms over time, others may face chronic challenges that affect their daily functioning and quality of life. Understanding these outcomes is crucial for families and healthcare providers alike, as it informs long-term management strategies and support systems.

One critical aspect to consider is the role of early intervention in shaping long-term outcomes. Studies suggest that those who receive prompt and appropriate treatment often fare better in the long run. Early warning signs, when recognised and acted upon, can lead to more effective treatment plans that not only address immediate symptoms but also promote recovery and stability. This reinforces the importance of public awareness and education regarding the early indicators of schizophrenia.

Another significant factor is the presence of co-occurring disorders, which can complicate the treatment process and influence long-term prognoses. Many individuals with schizophrenia may also struggle with substance abuse anxiety, or depressive disorders, further impacting their ability to engage in treatment and maintain a stable life. Addressing these co-occurring conditions through integrated treatment approaches is essential for improving overall outcomes and enhancing the quality of life.

Family support plays a pivotal role in the long-term management of schizophrenia. A strong support network can provide emotional and practical assistance, helping individuals navigate the complexities of their condition. Families that are educated about schizophrenia and actively involved in the treatment process can significantly enhance their loved one's recovery journey, reducing feelings of isolation and stigma that often accompany the disorder.

In conclusion, the long-term outcomes of schizophrenia are influenced by a combination of treatment, early intervention, support systems, and the presence of co-occurring disorders. By fostering a more informed and supportive environment, we can help individuals with schizophrenia achieve better life outcomes. Continued research into innovative treatment options and coping strategies remains imperative to address the evolving needs of this population, ultimately aiming for a more hopeful future for those affected by this condition.

9

Chapter 9: Innovations in Schizophrenia Research

Recent Advances in Understanding

Recent research has significantly advanced our understanding of schizophrenia, shedding light on its complex nature and the biological underpinnings that contribute to its onset. Studies have revealed that genetic factors play a crucial role in the development of schizophrenia, with specific genes linked to the disorder. Additionally, neuroimaging techniques have provided insights into the brain structures and functions that may be altered in individuals with schizophrenia, highlighting the importance of biological research in understanding this mental health condition.

Furthermore, the identification of early warning signs of schizophrenia has improved significantly, enabling earlier intervention and treatment. Researchers have been focusing on subtle changes in behaviour and cognition that may precede the onset of full-blown symptoms. By recognising these signs, families and healthcare providers can implement preventative strategies, which may mitigate the severity of the disorder and enhance the quality of life for those at risk.

Innovations in treatment options have also emerged, combining traditional therapeutic approaches with novel interventions. Cognitive behavioural therapy (CBT) remains a cornerstone of treatment; however, recent advances include the use of virtual reality and digital platforms to enhance therapeutic engagement. Moreover, pharmacological research has expanded beyond antipsychotics, exploring the potential of new medications that target various neurotransmitter systems, aiming to reduce side effects and improve efficacy.

Understanding the interplay between schizophrenia and co-occurring disorders has become an essential area of study. Many individuals diagnosed with schizophrenia also experience conditions such as anxiety, depression, or substance use disorders. By addressing these co-occurring issues in treatment plans, practitioners can provide more holistic care that caters to the individual's overall mental health needs, rather than focusing solely on schizophrenia.

Lastly, the role of family support in managing schizophrenia cannot be overstated. Recent findings suggest that families who are educated about the disorder and actively involved in the treatment process can significantly affect the recovery trajectory of their loved ones. Reducing stigma and misconceptions surrounding schizophrenia is vital in fostering a supportive environment for individuals affected by the disorder, allowing them to thrive in their daily lives and achieve better outcomes.

New Treatment Modalities

In recent years, the landscape of schizophrenia treatment has evolved significantly, introducing new modalities that aim to enhance the quality of life for individuals living with this condition. These innovations are pivotal, particularly considering the diverse experiences of those affected by schizophrenia, which can vary widely from one person to another. As researchers continue to explore the complexities of the disorder, they are developing treatment protocols that address not only the symptoms but also the underlying causes and co-occurring disorders that often accompany schizophrenia.

One promising area of development is the use of personalised medicine, which tailors treatment plans to the unique genetic, biological, and environmental factors of each individual. Such an approach can lead to more effective outcomes as it allows clinicians to select medications and therapies that are more likely to work for specific patients based on their unique profiles. This shift towards personalised care represents a significant departure from the traditional one-size-fits-all approach, which has often resulted in trial and error in medication management.

Another exciting advancement is the integration of technology into treatment strategies, such as the use of mobile applications and telehealth services. These tools enable individuals to access support and resources more readily, fostering a sense of connection and community that can be vital for those navigating the challenges of schizophrenia. Furthermore, technology can assist in monitoring symptoms and medication adherence, providing both patients and healthcare providers with valuable data to inform treatment decisions.

Psychosocial interventions have also seen a resurgence in interest as part of a holistic approach to managing schizophrenia. Techniques such as cognitive behavioural therapy (CBT) and family therapy are being adapted to cater specifically to the needs of individuals with schizophrenia and their families. These therapies not only focus on symptom management but also on enhancing coping strategies and improving the overall functioning of individuals, helping them to lead more fulfilling lives.

Finally, ongoing research into novel pharmacological agents continues to hold promise for the future of schizophrenia treatment. Investigations into new compounds that target different neurotransmitter systems are paving the way for more effective and tolerable medications. As these new treatment modalities come to fruition, they bring hope for improved outcomes and a better quality of life for those affected by schizophrenia, along with a deeper understanding of the disorder itself.

Future Directions in Research

As we look towards the future of research in schizophrenia, it is essential to recognise the importance of understanding the early warning signs of this complex disorder. Advances in neuroimaging and genetic studies are enabling researchers to identify biomarkers that may predict the onset of schizophrenia. This could lead to earlier interventions, which are crucial for improving outcomes and potentially preventing the full-blown manifestation of the disorder. By focusing on these early indicators, researchers aim to enhance the quality of life for individuals at risk of developing schizophrenia.

Moreover, the exploration of treatment options is evolving rapidly, with a growing emphasis on personalised medicine. Future research will likely delve into tailoring treatments based on individual genetic profiles and specific symptoms, rather than adopting a one-size-fits-all approach. This would not only improve the efficacy of treatments but also reduce side effects, making management of schizophrenia more sustainable. The integration of pharmacological and psychosocial interventions will remain a focal point in this personalised approach, ensuring a holistic treatment strategy.

Another critical area for future research is the relationship between schizophrenia and co-occurring disorders. Understanding how these conditions interact can provide valuable insights into effective treatment strategies. Future studies will seek to unravel the complexities of dual diagnoses, focusing on integrated treatment approaches that address both schizophrenia and accompanying conditions such as anxiety or substance use disorders. This comprehensive understanding is vital for improving overall patient outcomes and enhancing the effectiveness of interventions.

Family support plays a pivotal role in the management of schizophrenia, and future research will continue to explore how familial dynamics impact treatment adherence and recovery. Investigating the most effective ways to engage families in the treatment process will be essential in reducing stigma and fostering a supportive environment for individuals with schizophrenia. Research will likely focus on developing resources and training for families to better understand the disorder, thereby enhancing their ability to support their loved ones effectively.

Finally, addressing the stigma surrounding schizophrenia remains a significant challenge for researchers. Future directions will likely involve public health campaigns and educational initiatives aimed at dispelling myths and misconceptions about the disorder. By fostering a better understanding of schizophrenia within communities, researchers hope to create a more supportive environment for those affected. This shift in societal attitudes is crucial for encouraging individuals to seek help and improving their overall quality of life.

10

Chapter 10: Coping Strategies for Individuals with Schizophrenia

Self-management Techniques

Self-management techniques are vital for individuals living with schizophrenia, as they empower patients to take an active role in their treatment and daily lives. These techniques often involve a combination of strategies that help manage symptoms, reduce stress, and improve overall well-being. By understanding the importance of self-management, individuals can better navigate the complexities of their condition and work towards achieving a more stable and fulfilling life.

One effective self-management technique is the development of a structured daily routine. Establishing a consistent schedule can provide a sense of stability and predictability, which is particularly beneficial for those experiencing the unpredictable nature of schizophrenia. Incorporating regular activities such as exercise, meal preparation, and social interactions can help in maintaining mental health and reducing feelings of isolation.

Mindfulness and relaxation techniques also play a significant role in self-management. Practices such as meditation, deep breathing exercises, and yoga can help individuals to stay grounded and reduce anxiety. These techniques not only assist in managing immediate symptoms but also promote long-term emotional resilience, allowing individuals to cope better with the challenges associated with their condition.

Support networks are another crucial aspect of self-management. Engaging with family, friends, and support groups can provide emotional backing and practical assistance. It is important for individuals to communicate their needs and experiences to their support network, fostering an environment of understanding and compassion. This behaviour can significantly alleviate the stigma surrounding schizophrenia and promote a more inclusive approach to mental health.

Lastly, educating oneself about schizophrenia and its treatment options is essential for effective self-management. Knowledge empowers individuals to make informed decisions regarding their health and treatment, enabling them to advocate for their needs. Furthermore, staying informed about the latest research and innovations in schizophrenia treatment can inspire hope and motivate individuals to pursue their recovery journey actively.

Building Resilience

Building resilience is a vital aspect of managing schizophrenia, both for individuals experiencing the condition and their families. Resilience can be understood as the ability to adapt and recover from adversity, and it plays a crucial role in coping with the challenges posed by schizophrenia. By fostering resilience, individuals can better navigate their daily lives, manage symptoms, and improve their overall well-being. This chapter will explore strategies for building resilience and highlight the importance of a supportive environment in this process.

One of the foundational elements of resilience is the development of effective coping strategies. Individuals with schizophrenia can benefit from learning techniques that help them manage stress and emotional turmoil. This may include mindfulness practices, cognitive behavioural therapy, and engaging in physical activities. By equipping themselves with these tools, individuals can gain a sense of control over their experiences and reduce feelings of helplessness that often accompany the disorder.

Family support is another critical factor in building resilience. Families play a pivotal role in the recovery process, providing emotional backing, understanding, and practical assistance. Open communication within the family can foster a sense of belonging and reduce feelings of isolation for the individual. Educating family members about schizophrenia can also dispel myths and misconceptions, allowing them to better support their loved ones and create a nurturing environment that encourages resilience.

Moreover, engaging with peer support groups can significantly enhance resilience. These groups provide a platform for individuals to share their experiences, learn from one another, and offer mutual encouragement. The sense of community and shared understanding can be profoundly empowering, helping individuals to realise they are not alone in their journey. Through these connections, they can build a network of support that bolsters their resilience.

Lastly, it is essential to recognise that building resilience is a continuous process. Individuals with schizophrenia may face setbacks, but with the right strategies and support systems in place, they can learn to bounce back and thrive. As we continue to advance in schizophrenia research and treatment options, fostering resilience remains a key component in improving the quality of life for those affected by this complex condition.

Support Networks

Support networks play a crucial role in the lives of individuals diagnosed with schizophrenia. These networks can include family, friends, healthcare professionals, and community resources, all of which contribute to the overall well-being and recovery of the individual. When a person is faced with the challenges of schizophrenia, having a strong support system can provide emotional comfort and practical assistance in navigating the complexities of the disorder.

Family members often serve as the first line of support, offering understanding and encouragement. Their involvement can significantly impact treatment adherence and recovery outcomes. By educating themselves about schizophrenia, families can reduce stigma and foster a more supportive environment, which is vital for the individual's mental health. Open communication within the family can also help in recognising early warning signs and managing crises effectively.

Friends and peer support groups are equally important, as they provide a sense of belonging and reduce feelings of isolation. Engaging with others who understand similar experiences can empower individuals to share coping strategies and successes. These interactions can enhance self-esteem and motivate individuals to pursue their treatment plans actively, reinforcing the idea that recovery is achievable.

Healthcare professionals, including therapists and psychiatrists, form an essential part of the support network. They not only offer clinical treatment but also guide families and friends in understanding the nuances of schizophrenia. Collaborative care that includes family education and support can lead to better management of the disorder and improve the quality of life for everyone involved.

Finally, community resources such as support groups, educational workshops, and rehabilitation services provide additional layers of support. They can offer practical assistance, such as housing and employment resources, which are crucial for independent living. By utilising these networks, individuals with schizophrenia can build resilience and enhance their ability to cope with daily challenges, ultimately leading to a more fulfilling life.

11

Chapter 11: The Stigma Surrounding Schizophrenia

Understanding Stigma

Stigma is a pervasive issue that affects individuals with schizophrenia and their families. It refers to the negative attitudes and beliefs that society holds towards those with mental health disorders. This stigma can lead to discrimination, social exclusion, and a reluctance to seek help. Understanding stigma is crucial for fostering empathy and support for individuals living with schizophrenia, as it can significantly impact their treatment and recovery journey.

The stigma surrounding schizophrenia often stems from misconceptions and a lack of understanding about the disorder. Many people equate schizophrenia with violence or unpredictability, leading to fear and avoidance. This misrepresentation is compounded by media portrayals that sensationalise mental illness, further entrenching harmful stereotypes. By educating ourselves about the realities of schizophrenia, we can begin to dismantle these misconceptions and promote a more compassionate perspective.

Another critical aspect of stigma is its internalisation by those affected.

Individuals with schizophrenia may internalise negative societal attitudes, leading to feelings of shame and low self-worth. This internalised stigma can hinder their willingness to engage in treatment and can exacerbate feelings of isolation. Support from family and friends becomes vital in counteracting these negative feelings, helping individuals recognise their value beyond their diagnosis.

Addressing stigma requires a collective effort from all sectors of society, including healthcare professionals, policymakers, and the general public. Advocacy for mental health awareness, inclusive education, and supportive policies can create an environment where individuals feel safe to seek help without fear of judgement. Family support plays a crucial role in this process, as understanding and acceptance from loved ones can significantly improve the mental health outcomes for those affected by schizophrenia.

Ultimately, combating stigma is not just about changing perceptions; it is about empowering individuals with schizophrenia to live fulfilling lives. By fostering an inclusive society that values mental health, we can help those affected by schizophrenia navigate their challenges more effectively. Encouraging open conversations about mental health can lead to greater acceptance and understanding, paving the way for better treatment and support options for everyone involved.

Impact of Stigma on Individuals

Stigma surrounding schizophrenia significantly impacts individuals diagnosed with the disorder, often leading to feelings of shame and isolation. This negative perception not only affects their self-esteem but also discourages them from seeking help and disclosing their condition to others. Many individuals may internalise these societal attitudes, resulting in a detrimental cycle where stigma exacerbates their mental health challenges.

Moreover, the impact of stigma extends beyond the individual to affect their families and support networks. Family members may also experience stigma, which can create a sense of alienation and conflict within the household. This strain can hinder the ability of families to provide the necessary support for their loved ones, ultimately affecting treatment outcomes and overall well-being.

In the workplace, stigma can lead to discrimination and exclusion, making it challenging for individuals with schizophrenia to find and maintain employment. Fear of being judged or ostracised may prevent them from applying for jobs or fully participating in workplace activities. This economic disadvantage further compounds their mental health struggles, creating a cycle of poverty and mental illness that is difficult to escape.

Educational settings are not exempt from the effects of stigma, as students with schizophrenia may face bullying or social exclusion from their peers. This can lead to increased anxiety and hinder their academic performance, perpetuating the stigma associated with their condition. Educational institutions must foster an inclusive environment to support these individuals and combat the misconceptions that fuel stigma.

Addressing the impact of stigma requires a collective effort to educate the public and promote understanding of schizophrenia. By challenging myths and misconceptions, society can create a more supportive environment that empowers individuals with schizophrenia to seek help and engage with their communities. Ultimately, reducing stigma is crucial for improving the quality of life for those affected by this disorder.

Strategies for Reducing Stigma

Reducing stigma surrounding schizophrenia is crucial for fostering a supportive environment for individuals affected by this condition. One effective strategy is promoting education and awareness about schizophrenia, which helps dispel myths and misconceptions. By informing the public about the realities of the disorder, including its symptoms and treatment options, we can create a more understanding society. This knowledge can empower individuals to speak openly about their experiences and seek help without fear of judgement.

Another important strategy is encouraging open conversations about mental health within families and communities. When people are willing to share their stories and experiences, it humanises the condition and fosters empathy. Support groups and community forums can serve as platforms for these discussions, allowing individuals to connect with others who have faced similar challenges. This sense of community can significantly reduce feelings of isolation and shame often associated with schizophrenia.

Advocacy plays a vital role in reducing stigma as well. Engaging with policymakers to promote mental health initiatives and legislation can lead to systemic changes that support individuals with schizophrenia. Advocacy groups can help amplify voices of those affected, ensuring their needs and concerns are addressed in public policy. This not only raises awareness but also encourages society to view mental health as a critical aspect of overall health.

Media representation also has a significant impact on stigma. Encouraging responsible and accurate portrayals of schizophrenia in films, television, and news media can challenge existing stereotypes. By showcasing real stories of individuals living with schizophrenia and their triumphs, media can help shift public perception. This approach not only informs viewers but also highlights the importance of empathy and compassion towards those with mental health disorders.

Lastly, fostering supportive environments in workplaces and educational institutions is essential. Implementing policies that promote mental health awareness and provide resources for individuals struggling with schizophrenia can create a culture of acceptance. Training staff and educators to recognise early warning signs and provide appropriate support can make a significant difference. These strategies collectively contribute to a society that is more informed, compassionate, and supportive of individuals with schizophrenia.

12

I. Executive Summary

This briefing document provides a comprehensive overview of schizophrenia, a complex mental health disorder affecting thought, feelings, and behavior. Drawing from various sources, it delves into the disorder's definition, neuroscience, historical perspectives, symptoms, early warning signs, and treatment options. A significant emphasis is placed on the crucial role of family support, the impact of co-occurring conditions, innovations in research, coping strategies, and the pervasive issue of stigma. Early diagnosis and intervention, alongside a multifaceted approach to treatment encompassing medication, psychotherapy, and strong support networks, are consistently highlighted as vital for improving outcomes and quality of life for individuals with schizophrenia.

13

II. Understanding Schizophrenia: Definition, Neuroscience, and Historical Context

A. Definition and Overview

Schizophrenia is a "complex and often misunderstood mental health disorder that affects how a person thinks, feels, and behaves." It is characterized by symptoms such as "delusions, hallucinations, disorganised thinking, and emotional dysregulation," which can significantly impair daily functioning. Onset typically occurs "in late adolescence or early adulthood," making early diagnosis and intervention "crucial." The disorder's impact extends beyond the individual, affecting "family members and caregivers as well."

B. Neuroscience of Schizophrenia

Neuroscience has significantly advanced the understanding of schizophrenia, identifying various neurological anomalies:

- **Structural Abnormalities:** Studies show "enlarged ventricles and reduced grey matter in specific regions," impacting cognitive and emotional regulation.

- **Neuroanatomical Changes:** Key regions affected include the "prefrontal cortex," integral for higher cognitive functions like decision-making and emotional regulation, and the "hippocampus," essential for memory formation. Both show "reduced volume and activity," contributing to cognitive deficits and memory impairment. "Disrupted pathways" between these areas exacerbate symptoms.
- **Neurochemical Underpinnings:** "Neurotransmitters, particularly dopamine and glutamate, play crucial roles."
- **Dopaminergic Pathways:** The "dopamine hypothesis suggests that an overactivity of dopamine transmission may lead to positive symptoms, such as hallucinations and delusions" (mesolimbic pathway). Conversely, "impairments in this circuit [mesocortical pathway] can lead to negative symptoms of schizophrenia, such as social withdrawal and apathy."
- **Glutamate and NMDA Receptor Dysfunction:** "Abnormalities in this system may contribute to the symptoms," with "an excess of glutamate in certain brain regions, leading to excitotoxicity" for positive symptoms, and "a deficiency in NMDA receptor function...linked to the negative symptoms."
- **Inflammation and Immune System:** "Microglia," the brain's immune cells, can become "overactive, leading to chronic inflammation." Elevated "pro-inflammatory cytokines" can disrupt neurotransmitter systems, contributing to "hallucinations and cognitive dysfunction."
- **Genetics and Epigenetics:** Schizophrenia has a "heritable component," with "multiple genes" contributing to susceptibility. "Environmental influences can affect gene expression" through epigenetic modifications, where factors like "stress, trauma, and substance abuse" can trigger or exacerbate symptoms in genetically predisposed individuals.
- **Risk Genes:** Specific genes implicated include "DISC1" (neural development, synaptic transmission), "COMT" (dopamine metabolism), and the "22q11.2 deletion syndrome" (a significant genetic risk factor disrupting multiple genes).
- **Heritability and Gene-Environment Interaction:** Schizophrenia is not solely determined by genetics but by a "complex interplay of both inher-

ited traits and environmental influences." Early life experiences can also influence development.

- **Brain Imaging and Biomarkers:** Techniques like "MRI" (Magnetic Resonance Imaging) and "PET" (Positron Emission Tomography) reveal "structural abnormalities, such as enlarged ventricles and reduced grey matter," and altered "metabolic activity" respectively. "Biomarkers" are sought to "predict the onset of schizophrenia or the likelihood of a particular treatment being effective."
- **Functional Connectivity Disruptions:** These refer to "alterations in the communication pathways between different regions of the brain," contributing to cognitive and perceptual disturbances. Key areas like the "prefrontal cortex" and the "default mode network" show abnormal connectivity.

C. Historical Perspectives

The understanding of schizophrenia has evolved significantly:

- **Ancient Civilizations:** Symptoms were attributed to "spiritual or supernatural forces, viewing those affected as possessed or cursed."
- **Emil Kraepelin (German Psychiatrist):** In the 19th century, Kraepelin "laid the groundwork for recognising schizophrenia as a distinct illness," emphasizing its "biological underpinnings" and classifying different forms.
- **Eugen Bleuler (Swiss Psychiatrist):** In the early 20th century, Bleuler coined the term "schizophrenia" (splitting of the mind) and identified "four fundamental symptoms: affective blunting, autism, ambivalence, and associative looseness." He also emphasized "early intervention" and the "significant impact of social and familial support."
- **Sigmund Freud (Neurologist, Psychoanalyst):** Proposed that schizophrenia arises from "unresolved conflicts within the psyche, particularly involving the unconscious mind." While his theories have faced criticism for overshadowing biological factors, his focus on "early childhood

experiences" and "personal history" influenced holistic therapeutic practices.

- **Carl Jung (Swiss Psychiatrist and Psychoanalyst):** Viewed schizophrenia through the "lens of archetypes and the collective unconscious," believing symptoms could reveal "unresolved issues within the individual's unconscious mind." He also emphasized the importance of a "supportive and understanding environment."
- **Eric Kandel (Nobel Prize-winning Neuroscientist):** His work on "molecular mechanisms that underlie synaptic plasticity" is highly relevant, as "disruptions in these mechanisms may contribute to the cognitive deficits."
- **Iain McGilchrist (Neuropsychiatrist):** Suggests schizophrenia may be a "disruption in the balance of these hemispheric functions," with a left hemisphere dominance leading to a "narrowed focus on details at the expense of broader contextual understanding."

14

III. Symptoms, Early Warning Signs, and Treatment Options

A. Symptoms and Types

Common symptoms include "hallucinations, delusions, disorganised thinking, and impaired functioning."

- **Hallucinations:** "hearing voices or seeing things that are not present."
- **Delusions:** "firmly held false beliefs that can lead to paranoia or significant misinterpretations of reality."
- **Types:** Include "paranoid schizophrenia" (intense paranoia, auditory hallucinations), "disorganised schizophrenia" (disorganised speech and behaviour), and "catatonic schizophrenia" (motor behaviour ranging from agitation to immobility).

B. Early Warning Signs

"Recognising the early symptoms of schizophrenia is crucial for effective intervention." These can be subtle and include:

- **Behavioural Changes:** "withdrawal from social interactions, a decline in academic or work performance, and an unusual preoccupation with certain thoughts or beliefs." Also, "alteration in daily routines and self-care practices," and "inappropriate or exaggerated reactions to situations."
- **Perceptual Disturbances:** "hearing voices or seeing things that others do not."
- **Emotional State:** "anxiety, depression, or sudden mood swings."
- "Co-occurring disorders, such as substance abuse or anxiety disorders," can complicate early recognition.

C. Treatment Options

Treatment is "diverse and often include a combination of medication, psychotherapy, and support services."

- **Medication Approaches:** "Antipsychotic medications are commonly prescribed to manage symptoms," targeting neurotransmitter systems like dopamine. "Newer atypical antipsychotics" offer different mechanisms and potentially fewer side effects.
- **Psychotherapy and Supportive Therapies:** "Cognitive-behavioural therapy (CBT)" helps identify and challenge "distorted thought patterns." "Supportive therapies, such as group therapy and family therapy," provide community and understanding.
- **Holistic and Alternative Treatments:** Complement traditional approaches by focusing on "physical, emotional, and spiritual well-being." Examples include "mindfulness and meditation" and "nutritional therapies" (e.g., omega-3 fatty acids).

15

IV. Schizophrenia and Co-occurring Disorders

A. Common Co-occurring Conditions

Schizophrenia is frequently accompanied by other conditions, complicating diagnosis and treatment.

- **Mood Disorders:** "depression and bipolar disorder" can intensify feelings of hopelessness.
- **Anxiety Disorders:** "excessive worry, panic attacks, or social anxiety" can lead to further isolation.
- **Substance Use Disorders:** Often used as "self-medication," these can worsen symptoms and hinder treatment adherence.

B. Impact on Treatment and Management

Co-occurring disorders necessitate "integrated management strategies." "Effective management requires a combination of medication, therapy, and support, all tailored to the unique needs."

C. Integrated Treatment Strategies

Focus on a "comprehensive approach" combining "pharmacological treatments with psychosocial interventions."

- **Collaboration:** "Psychiatrists, psychologists, social workers, and occupational therapists often work as a cohesive team."
- **Holistic Approach:** Addresses "mental, emotional, and social needs," as well as co-occurring disorders.

16

V. The Role of Family Support in Schizophrenia Management

A. Importance of Family Involvement

"Family involvement plays a crucial role in the management and understanding of schizophrenia." Families are often the "first line of support, recognising early warning signs and providing essential emotional and practical assistance." This involvement "aids in symptom management" and fosters "a sense of belonging and understanding."

B. Effective Communication Strategies

"Clear and open dialogue" is critical.

- **Active Listening:** "giving full attention...acknowledging their feelings, and validating their experiences."
- **Clear and Concise Language:** Avoiding "jargon and technical terms" and using "visual aids or written materials."
- **Non-verbal Communication:** "Body language, facial expressions, and tone of voice can convey empathy and understanding."

C. Support Resources for Families

Families need resources like "educational materials, workshops, and support groups" from mental health organizations. "Professional resources" like therapists and counselors, and "advocacy groups," are also vital. Families must also "prioritise their own mental health and well-being."

17

VI. Schizophrenia Myths and Misconceptions

A. Common Misconceptions

- **Split Personality:** "individuals with schizophrenia have a split personality or are simply 'mad'." This is inaccurate; it's distinct from dissociative identity disorder.
- **Violence:** "individuals with schizophrenia are dangerous." Research shows they are "more likely to be victims of violence rather than perpetrators."
- **Rarity:** "schizophrenia is a rare disorder," when it affects "approximately 1 in 100 people worldwide."
- **Adult-only Onset:** "schizophrenia only occurs in adults." It can manifest in "adolescence."
- **Untreatable:** "there is no effective treatment available." Advances have led to "various treatment modalities...that can help manage symptoms effectively."

B. The Reality of Schizophrenia

It is a complex condition with varying symptoms and onset. "The stigma surrounding it" is a major challenge, leading to "discrimination and misunderstanding." "Recovery is possible" with "the right treatment and support."

C. Educating Others

"Educating others about schizophrenia is crucial in dispelling myths and misconceptions." This can be done through "community workshops and seminars," "social media and online platforms," and by "fostering supportive environments in workplaces and educational institutions."

18

VII. Impact of Schizophrenia on Daily Life

A. Challenges in Daily Functioning

Individuals struggle with tasks like "maintaining personal hygiene, adhering to medication schedules, or managing daily responsibilities."

- **Cognitive Difficulties:** "Problems with attention, memory, and executive functioning."
- **Social Interactions:** "paranoia or delusions that make it challenging to engage with others, leading to social withdrawal."
- Co-occurring disorders further complicate daily functioning.

B. Social Relationships and Community Integration

"Supportive friendships and community ties can help mitigate feelings of isolation." "Family support is particularly significant." "Community integration initiatives" like social skills training and peer support reduce stigma and promote acceptance.

C. Employment and Education Considerations

Individuals face challenges in "maintaining stable employment and pursuing educational opportunities."

- **Flexible Employment Options:** "Job accommodations, such as flexible hours or remote work opportunities."
- **Supportive Educational Settings:** "access to mental health resources on campus, as well as academic accommodations."
- Family support is crucial in navigating these challenges.

19

VIII. Schizophrenia in Adolescents vs. Adults

A. Differences in Onset and Symptoms

Onset can be "gradual over months or years" or "sudden." Symptoms vary widely. In "adolescents, the onset of schizophrenia often coincides with significant developmental changes," leading to symptoms being "mistaken for typical teenage behaviour."

B. Treatment Approaches for Different Age Groups

- **Children and Adolescents:** Focus on "education, therapy, and family involvement" within a "supportive environment."
- **Adults:** Typically involves "pharmacological interventions and psychotherapy" (CBT).
- **Older Adults:** Requires "adjustments to medication and increased focus on psychosocial support."

C. Long-term Outcomes

Vary significantly based on "severity...age of onset, and the availability of treatment options." "Early intervention" leads to better outcomes. Co-occurring disorders complicate prognoses. "Family support plays a pivotal role."

20

IX. Innovations in Schizophrenia Research

A. Recent Advances in Understanding

- **Genetic Factors:** "crucial role in the development."
- **Neuroimaging Techniques:** "insights into the brain structures and functions that may be altered."
- **Early Warning Signs:** "subtle changes in behaviour and cognition."

B. New Treatment Modalities

- **Personalised Medicine:** "tailors treatment plans to the unique genetic, biological, and environmental factors of each individual."
- **Technology Integration:** "mobile applications and telehealth services" for support and symptom monitoring.
- **Psychosocial Interventions:** Adaptations of CBT and family therapy.
- **Novel Pharmacological Agents:** Targeting different neurotransmitter systems for more effective and tolerable medications.

C. Future Directions in Research

- **Early Interventions:** Identifying biomarkers for prediction and prevention.
- **Personalised Medicine:** Tailoring treatments based on genetic profiles and specific symptoms.
- **Co-occurring Disorders:** Understanding their interaction and developing integrated treatment approaches.
- **Family Support:** Exploring effective ways to engage families and provide resources.
- **Reducing Stigma:** Public health campaigns and educational initiatives.

21

X. Coping Strategies for Individuals with Schizophrenia

A. Self-management Techniques

Empower patients to take an active role.

- **Structured Daily Routine:** "consistency...stability and predictability."
- **Mindfulness and Relaxation:** "meditation, deep breathing exercises, and yoga."
- **Support Networks:** "Engaging with family, friends, and support groups."
- **Education:** "educating oneself about schizophrenia and its treatment options."

B. Building Resilience

"the ability to adapt and recover from adversity."

- **Effective Coping Strategies:** Managing stress and emotional turmoil.
- **Family Support:** "emotional backing, understanding, and practical assistance."

- **Peer Support Groups:** "sense of community and shared understanding."
- Recognizing that "building resilience is a continuous process."

C. Support Networks

Crucial for "overall well-being and recovery."

- **Family Members:** "first line of support," impacting treatment adherence and reducing stigma.
- **Friends and Peer Support Groups:** "sense of belonging and reduce feelings of isolation."
- **Healthcare Professionals:** Provide clinical treatment and guidance.
- **Community Resources:** Support groups, educational workshops, rehabilitation services.

22

XI. Conclusion: Combating Stigma and Fostering Support

Across all aspects of schizophrenia, the consistent themes of **early intervention, multifaceted treatment, strong family support, and active efforts to combat stigma** are paramount. The journey with schizophrenia is complex, but with informed care, understanding, and a supportive environment, individuals can manage their symptoms, build resilience, and lead fulfilling lives. Ongoing research and education are essential to continue advancing treatment and fostering a more empathetic society for those affected by this condition.

23

FAQ

1. What is schizophrenia and how does it manifest?

Schizophrenia is a complex mental health disorder that profoundly impacts how an individual thinks, feels, and behaves. It is characterized by a range of symptoms, including positive symptoms like **delusions** (firmly held false beliefs) and **hallucinations** (perceiving things that aren't real, often auditory or visual). Other key manifestations include **disorganized thinking** and speech, **emotional dysregulation** (affective blunting), **social withdrawal** (autism), **apathy**, and **lack of motivation** (negative symptoms). The onset typically occurs in late adolescence or early adulthood, though it can appear at any age. Early warning signs can include subtle changes in behavior like social withdrawal, declines in academic or work performance, unusual preoccupations, mood swings, anxiety, and neglecting self-care. There are different types, such as paranoid schizophrenia (characterized by paranoia and hallucinations), disorganized schizophrenia (marked by disorganized speech and behavior), and catatonic schizophrenia (involving extreme motor agitation or immobility).

2. What are the key neurobiological insights into schizophrenia?

Neuroscience has significantly advanced our understanding of schizophrenia, identifying various neurological anomalies and neurochemical imbalances. Individuals with schizophrenia often exhibit **structural abnormalities** in the brain, such as enlarged ventricles and reduced grey matter in regions like the **prefrontal cortex** (affecting cognitive functions, decision-making, and emotional regulation) and the **hippocampus** (linked to memory and learning difficulties).

Neurochemically, the disorder is strongly linked to dysfunction in neurotransmitter systems, particularly **dopamine** and **glutamate**. The **dopamine hypothesis** suggests an overactivity of dopamine in the mesolimbic pathway contributes to positive symptoms like hallucinations and delusions, while underactivity in the mesocortical pathway is linked to negative symptoms and cognitive deficits. **Glutamatergic dysfunction**, specifically involving **NMDA receptors**, is also implicated in both cognitive deficits and altered perception.

Recent advances in **neuroimaging techniques** like fMRI and PET scans reveal altered brain connectivity and activity patterns, highlighting how disrupted brain networks contribute to psychosis. Additionally, research points to the role of **inflammation and the immune system**, with **microglial activation** and elevated pro-inflammatory cytokines potentially contributing to symptoms and affecting treatment efficacy.

3. How do genetics and environment interact in the development of schizophrenia?

Schizophrenia has a strong **heritable component**, meaning genetic factors significantly contribute to an individual's susceptibility. Family and twin studies indicate that the disorder is influenced by multiple genes, not just one, with individuals having a family history being at higher risk. However, genetic predisposition alone does not guarantee onset.

Epigenetics explains how environmental influences can affect gene expression, even in genetically predisposed individuals. Factors such as **stress,**

trauma, and substance abuse can lead to epigenetic modifications that may trigger or exacerbate symptoms. This highlights a dynamic **gene-environment interaction**, where inherited risks combine with external factors to influence whether schizophrenia develops. Specific "risk genes" like **DISC1** (involved in neural development), **COMT** (affecting dopamine metabolism), and the **22q11.2 deletion syndrome** (a significant genetic risk factor) further illustrate the biological underpinnings and how genetic vulnerabilities can interact with environmental triggers.

4. What are the primary treatment approaches for schizophrenia?

Treatment for schizophrenia typically involves a **multifaceted approach** combining various strategies for optimal outcomes. **Medication approaches** are a cornerstone, with **antipsychotic medications** commonly prescribed to manage symptoms by altering neurotransmitter levels, especially dopamine. Both traditional and newer atypical antipsychotics are used, with careful monitoring for side effects. **Psychotherapy and supportive therapies** are crucial complements. **Cognitive Behavioral Therapy (CBT)** helps individuals challenge distorted thoughts and develop coping strategies. **Supportive therapies** like group therapy and family therapy provide a sense of community, reduce isolation, and foster open communication among family members to better understand and support their loved ones. **Holistic and alternative treatments** are also gaining recognition, focusing on overall well-being. These can include mindfulness, meditation, and nutritional therapies, which may help manage stress, anxiety, and support brain health, complementing conventional treatments. Integrated treatment strategies emphasize collaboration among different healthcare professionals and addressing co-occurring disorders.

5. Why is early intervention important in managing schizophrenia?

Early intervention is crucial for improving long-term outcomes and enhancing the quality of life for individuals with schizophrenia. Recognizing early warning signs—such as social withdrawal, changes in mood, unusual thoughts, or declines in functioning—allows for **timely treatment and support**.

When intervention occurs at an early stage, it can significantly **reduce the severity of symptoms** and their impact on daily functioning, leading to a more favorable prognosis. Early detection also plays a vital role in **preventing the development of co-occurring disorders** like substance abuse, depression, or anxiety, which often complicate the course of schizophrenia. By addressing these issues concurrently, individuals are more likely to achieve better overall mental health outcomes. Early intervention also considers that neurobiological changes in the brain can occur before full psychotic symptoms, paving the way for preventative strategies and potentially altering the illness's trajectory.

6. What is the role of family support in schizophrenia management?

Family support is **crucial and multifaceted** in the management of schizophrenia. Families often serve as the **first line of support**, being the first to recognize early warning signs and providing essential emotional and practical assistance. Their active involvement significantly **impacts overall treatment outcomes**, as studies show patients are more likely to adhere to treatment regimens when families participate in planning and decision-making.

Families can **educate themselves** about the disorder, dispelling myths and misconceptions, which in turn **reduces stigma** and fosters a more supportive home environment. Effective communication strategies, including active listening and clear language, are vital for building trust and providing a safe space for individuals to express themselves. Beyond practical support, families provide emotional backing, reducing feelings of isolation and distress, and helping individuals develop coping strategies and rebuild confidence. Support resources for families, such as educational materials, workshops, and support groups, further empower them to navigate the complexities of caring for a loved one with schizophrenia.

7. What are common myths and misconceptions about schizophrenia, and how can they be addressed?

Common misconceptions about schizophrenia are widespread and contribute significantly to stigma. A major myth is that individuals with schizophrenia have a **"split personality"** or are inherently violent. This is inaccurate; schizophrenia does not involve multiple distinct identities, and those with the disorder are statistically more likely to be victims of violence than perpetrators. Another misconception is that schizophrenia is rare or only affects adults, when in fact, it impacts approximately 1 in 100 people worldwide and can manifest in adolescence, with early signs often mistaken for typical teenage behavior. There's also a misconception that there are no effective treatments, despite advances in medication and psychotherapy.

These myths can be addressed through various **strategies for reducing stigma**:

- **Education and awareness campaigns** are crucial for dispelling false beliefs and providing accurate information about symptoms, realities, and treatment options.
- **Encouraging open conversations** about mental health within families and communities humanizes the condition and fosters empathy.
- **Advocacy** for mental health initiatives and policies helps create systemic change and ensure adequate resources.
- **Responsible media representation** that showcases real stories and challenges stereotypes can significantly shift public perception.
- Fostering **supportive environments** in workplaces and educational institutions through policies and resources promotes acceptance and inclusiv-

ity.

8. How does schizophrenia impact an individual's daily life, and what considerations are there for different age groups?

Schizophrenia significantly impacts an individual's daily life, affecting **daily functioning, social relationships, employment, and education**. Individuals often struggle with basic self-care, maintaining routines, and managing responsibilities due to **cognitive difficulties** (attention, memory, executive functioning) and symptoms like **paranoia or disorganization**. This can lead to social withdrawal, isolation, and strained relationships. The presence of **co-occurring disorders** (like depression or substance abuse) further complicates daily life and treatment.

For adolescents, the onset of schizophrenia often coincides with significant developmental changes, and symptoms may be mistaken for typical teenage behavior, leading to delays in diagnosis. Early intervention in this group is crucial, focusing on education, therapy, and family involvement to create a supportive environment.

Adults typically receive treatment combining medication and psychotherapy, with a focus on coping strategies and community resources.

Older adults may face unique challenges due to comorbidities and potential cognitive decline, requiring adjusted medication and increased psychosocial support. Across all age groups, a holistic, tailored approach that recognizes age-related differences, addresses co-occurring conditions, and integrates strong family and community support is essential for improving overall quality of life and empowering individuals to lead fulfilling lives despite the challenges.

24

📚 Books

🔬 Medical & Neuroscience Focus

1. **"Surviving Schizophrenia: A Family Manual"** – *E. Fuller Torrey*

- Classic, practical guide written by a psychiatrist for families and patients.

1. **"The Neuroscience of Schizophrenia"** – *Anthony Grace & David Lewis*

- A professional reference exploring brain mechanisms and pathways involved.

1. **"Schizophrenia: A Very Short Introduction"** – *Chris Frith & Eve Johnstone*

- Concise and accessible introduction to the science and symptoms.

1. **"The Center Cannot Hold: My Journey Through Madness"** – *Elyn Saks*

- A memoir by a law professor with schizophrenia. Insightful, moving, and educational.

1. **"Is There No Place on Earth for Me?"** – *Susan Sheehan*

- Pulitzer Prize-winning book following the story of a woman living with schizophrenia in NYC.

25

Academic Articles & Reviews

Key Reviews and Meta-Analyses:

1. **Insel TR. (2010). "Rethinking Schizophrenia."***Nature, 468(7321), 187–193.*https://doi.org/10.1038/nature09552

- Landmark paper by the former NIMH director calling for a new neurobiological framework.

1. **Tandon R et al. (2013). "Schizophrenia, 'just the facts' what we know in 2013."***Schizophrenia Research, 150(1):3–13.*https://doi.org/10.1016/j.schres.2013.05.004

- Comprehensive update on causes, symptoms, and treatment.

1. **van Os J, Kapur S. (2009). "Schizophrenia."***The Lancet, 374(9690), 635–645.*https://doi.org/10.1016/S0140-6736(09)60995-8

- Focus on pathophysiology, dopamine, and diagnostic frameworks.

26

🌐 Websites

Trusted Institutions

1. **National Institute of Mental Health (NIMH)**https://www.nimh.nih.gov/health/topics/schizophrenia

- Government-funded source with accessible info on symptoms, treatment, and research.

1. **Schizophrenia and Related Disorders Alliance of America (SARDAA)** https://sardaa.org

- Advocacy, peer support groups, educational tools.

1. **Royal College of Psychiatrists (UK)**https://www.rcpsych.ac.uk/mental-health/problems-disorders/schizophrenia

- Patient and clinician education with downloadable leaflets.

1. **Mind Australia** *(for Australian context)*https://www.mindaustralia.org.au

- Support services, treatment info, family resources.

1. **Psychology Today – Schizophrenia**https://www.psychologytoday.com/intl/conditions/schizophrenia

- Useful articles, blogs, and patient-centered content.

www.ingramcontent.com/pod-product-compliance
Lightning Source LLC
LaVergne TN
LVHW090422210926
848480LV00002B/651
* 9 7 9 8 2 3 2 7 8 0 5 6 2 *